Betrayal & Beyond

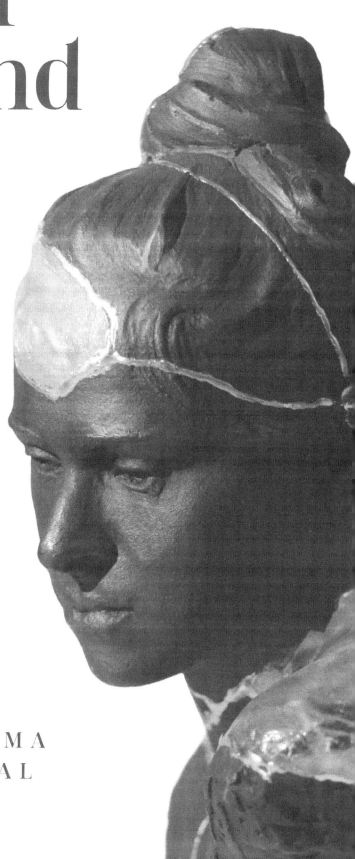

HEALING THE TRAUMA OF SEXUAL BETRAYAL

BETRAYAL & BEYOND WORKBOOK

By Diane Roberts

Other contributing writers:
Ted Roberts, Jane Carter, Teri Vietti, and Elizabeth Drago
2022 Version: Heather Kolb and Ashley Jameson

Copyright © 2016 by Ted & Diane Roberts

Copyright © 2020, 2022 by Pure Desire Ministries Intl.

All rights reserved. This book or parts thereof may not be reproduced in any form, stored in a retrieval system, or transmitted in any form by any means—electronic, mechanical, photocopy, recording, or otherwise—without prior written permission of Pure Desire Ministries International, except as provided by United States of America copyright law.

Published by
Pure Desire Ministries International
886 NW Corporate Dr, Troutdale, OR 97060
www.puredesire.org | 503.489.0230

ISBN 978-1-943291-18-2

The stories presented of individual lives in this Journal are true and accurate. The details have been adjusted to prevent personal identification. In some cases the story presented is a compilation of the histories of several individuals. The compilation, however, doesn't affect the clinical or theological veracity of the stories.

Scripture taken from the Holy Bible, NEW INTERNATIONAL VERSION®, NIV® Copyright © 1973, 1978, 1984, 2011 by Biblica, Inc.® Used by permission. All rights reserved worldwide.

Scripture quotations are taken from the Holy Bible, New Living Translation, copyright ©1996, 2004, 2007, 2013, 2015 by Tyndale House Foundation. Used by permission of Tyndale House Publishers, Inc., Carol Stream, Illinois 60188. All rights reserved.

Scripture quotations from THE MESSAGE. Copyright © by Eugene H. Peterson 1993, 1994, 1995, 1996, 2000, 2001, 2002. Used by permission of NavPress. All rights reserved. Represented by Tyndale House Publishers, Inc.

Scripture taken from the New King James Version®. Copyright © 1982 by Thomas Nelson. Used by permission. All rights reserved.

Scripture quotations marked (TLB) are taken from The Living Bible copyright © 1971. Used by permission of Tyndale House Publishers, Inc., Carol Stream, Illinois 60188. All rights reserved.

Content editing by Heather Kolb

Copy editing by Sue Miholer

Cover design and interior design by Elisabeth Windsor

Typesetting by Elisabeth Windsor, Emily Park, Justin Watson, and Trevor Winsor

Dump truck illustration by Sarah Peters

Betrayal
& Beyond

HEALING THE TRAUMA
OF SEXUAL BETRAYAL

Based on the original work of Diane Roberts

New and updated version written by Heather Kolb and Ashley Jameson

Contents

Acknowledgments

Pure Desire Ministries wishes to acknowledge the following contributors:

We are so grateful for the foundational work of Diane Roberts, cofounder of Pure Desire Ministries. *Betrayal & Beyond* was created from her extensive experience with helping partners and couples heal from the pain of sexual brokenness and betrayal trauma. Her years of clinical expertise, walking with couples through the process of restoration, is what gives us a glimpse into the real life stories shared throughout this material. Thank you, Diane, for your heart and passion for partners, that they would find lasting healing from betrayal; and your dedication to couples, that through recovery and healing, they would experience a life and marriage exceedingly blessed by God.

During this process, we were blessed to receive feedback and suggestions from Dr. Barbara Steffens, a leading expert on betrayal trauma and cofounder of APSATS (Association of Partners of Sex Addicts Trauma Specialists). It was through her continued support and encouragement that we were able to create this partner sensitive, trauma informed resource for betrayed partners. Dr. Steffens, we are forever grateful for your soft spoken encouragement and for the times you said, "You might want to say…" Thank you for your obvious heart for partners and for creating a method that empowers partners to thrive on their healing journey.

In many ways, this update to *Betrayal & Beyond* was prompted by Ashley Jameson, Associate Director of Women's Groups for Pure Desire. When it comes to Pure Desire groups, she is on the front line, having thousands of conversations with women about what makes the material work and what could make it better. She encouraged women to give feedback and she listened. Ashley, your passion for helping others heal is contagious. Thank you for reflecting Jesus, not only in your tenacity to bring about positive change but in your genuine love for people. This update would not have happened without you.

As the Content Manager for Pure Desire, Heather Kolb has spent months writing and rewriting, reorganizing, and writing more to ensure this resource takes a partner sensitive approach to healing from betrayal trauma. Building on what makes Pure Desire unique, she used science and statistical data, and laid it over a foundation of biblical truth. Thank you, Heather, for your extensive work on *Betrayal & Beyond*. Your willingness to stand in the gap for partners and create a more trauma informed approach, reveals your heart and sensitivity toward those who have been wounded through betrayal. Thank you for making this update a reality.

Most importantly, thank you heavenly Father for continuing to inspire and bless this work, bringing hope, healing, and freedom to those impacted by betrayal trauma. None of this would be possible without Your divine guidance and grace. Lord, for all the women who have experienced betrayal, will You comfort their broken hearts and bring them healing as only You can do.

Introduction

The day of discovery will likely be one you never forget. In some cases, maybe you've been aware of his struggle for a long time and it's finally come to a breaking point. Regardless of whether you were completely caught off guard or possibly suspected something was wrong, the magnitude of devastation is inconceivable. The life you thought you had is gone. The person you thought you married has been replaced with a stranger; someone who looks like your husband, but has hurt you in a way you never thought possible. And now, you are consumed with thoughts and feelings you've never experienced before—thoughts and feelings you can't even describe.

For many women who experience betrayal, it tends to have an accumulative effect. Much like a hurricane generates energy as it moves across the ocean,[1] so it is with the impact of betrayal. There is a growing, gradual increase in our pain. In our shock and disbelief. In our inability to make sense of what's happening. In our search for the truth. And in the trauma we're experiencing because of betrayal.

Jesus never said He would pull us out of the storms of life. Instead, He promised to be our anchor in the midst of the storm and walk with us through the storm. Isaiah 43:2 reveals God's commitment to us when we are experiencing the storms and pain of this life:

> *When you pass through the waters, I will be with you; And through the rivers, they shall not overflow you. When you walk through the fire, you shall not be burned, Nor shall the flame scorch you.*
>
> HEBREWS 6:19–20B (NIV)

This healing journey will help us walk in the tension of dealing honestly with our pain and trauma while holding onto Jesus as our anchor.

---

[1] Marshall Brain, Craig Freudenrich, and Robert Lamb, "How Hurricanes Work," HowStuffWorks, June 30, 2021, https://science.howstuffworks.com/nature/climate-weather/storms/hurricane-intensity-increasing.htm.

We often think of trauma as the actual incident or event that happened to us. But there's really more to it.

Trauma is a reaction of our bodies, minds, and emotions to a deeply distressing event. The earth-shattering incident changes the way we see people in our world and unravels our sense of safety. We can't go back. We can't erase what happened to us. Who we are and how we live significantly shift. Like a death, earthquake, or car crash, the event happens suddenly and changes us without warning, causing us to feel shock, denial, agony, terror, or helplessness.[2]

Trauma is the feeling we're left with after something happens to us.[3] The incident or event is traumatic. How it makes us feel and the feelings we take away from the incident or event, this is trauma. And the way we experience trauma, and how we are impacted by it, is specific to each of us.

With betrayal trauma there is a deeper level of complexity involved. According to Dr. Jennifer Freyd:

> 66 *Betrayal trauma occurs when the people or institutions on which a person depends for survival significantly violate that person's trust or well-being...[4]*

Betrayal trauma is unique. It involves someone we trust. Someone we depend on. Someone we are in a relationship with. And they have done something to violate our trust and, even more so, have caused us immeasurable pain.

Dr. Barbara Steffens, a leading expert in betrayal trauma, writes:

I think the most startling outcome of my study was that 70 percent of the women met the symptomatic criteria for PTSD in response to the disclosure of sexual addiction. This is not to say that they have PTSD, but that the level of symptoms is consistent with those in someone exposed to a natural disaster or sexual assault who went on to develop PTSD as a result of that event. To me, that is significant information for the spouse and for those who seek to help him or her heal.[5]

---

[2] Sheri Keffer, *Intimate Deception: Healing the Wounds of Sexual Betrayal* (Grand Rapids: Revell, 2018), 45.

[3] Craig Cashwell, PSAP Training Program,Module 2, Day 2, International Institute for Trauma & Addiction Professionals, Portland, Oregon, November 2, 2021.

[4] Freyd, J.J. (2021). *What is a Betrayal Trauma? What is Betrayal Trauma Theory?* Retrieved May 24, 2022 from http://pages.uoregon.edu/dynamic/jjf/defineBT.html.

[5] Barbara Steffens and Marsha Means, *Your Sexually Addicted Spouse: How Partners Can Cope and Heal* (Far Hills: New Horizon Press, 2009), 62.

Common symptoms experienced by a betrayed partner include (but are not limited to): shock, physical distress, sleep disturbances, changes in eating behaviors, emotional distress, hypervigilance, anxiety, stress, and intrusive thoughts.[6]

Perhaps you've experienced some of these symptoms. They are often the result of a significant, life-altering traumatic event. They are consistent among women who have experienced betrayal trauma.

Although betrayal has created so much pain and trauma in your life, we're so thankful you've chosen to get healing for yourself. Joining a support group, with other women who are on this same healing journey, is a great first step. Being able to process your experiences in a safe, grace-filled place—and working at a pace that encourages self-discovery—will empower you to make strides in your healing and equip you to make informed decisions for your future.

With a fresh perspective on trauma treatment, *Betrayal & Beyond* takes a partner sensitive approach to healing from the effects of sexual betrayal.

Throughout this study, you will:

- gain a greater understanding of how the trauma from betrayal is impacting your mind, body, and soul.
- apply strategies to keep you safe and emotionally healthy.
- identify and recognize the symptoms of trauma.
- incorporate proactive strategies to alleviate trauma symptoms during times of stress.
- learn the power of self-care.
- reestablish trust and emotional health in your relationship.
- create a plan for your future that is informed, intentional, and healthy.

All of this, and so much more, from a biblically based and clinically informed approach to healing!

Healing from sexual betrayal is a long journey—a journey no woman ever plans to take. But when we embrace this journey with God and others, it transforms who we are and empowers who we are becoming.

---

[6] Barbara A. Steffens and Robyn L. Rennie, "The Traumatic Nature of Disclosure for Wives of Sexual Addicts," *Sexual Addiction & Compulsivity*, 13:2-3, 247- 267, 2006, DOI: 10.1080/10720160600870802.

Weekly Expectations

The weekly lessons contain information to help you gain a greater understanding of betrayal trauma, become aware of how it is impacting your life, and give you the tools you need to find healing.

WORKBOOK LESSONS - OVERVIEW

The workbook lessons may consist of a variety of tasks: reading, assessments, answering questions, filling in tables, and more. Do your best to complete all the homework within each lesson. However, do not feel pressured to force an answer if you don't have one or you're not ready to give an answer.

Healing from betrayal trauma is a slow process. Although you have the support of this group to help you throughout this journey, this is really a journey of self-discovery. It's about you finding the answers you need, with the help of the Holy Spirit and the women in this group. This is about you taking ownership of your healing and being empowered to discover the life God has for you.

For partners who are single, separated, or divorced, do your best to answer the questions according to WHEN they happened, as they relate to the relationship in which you were betrayed. This will help you work through the pain and trauma you've experienced and find healing from it.

JOURNAL LESSONS - OVERVIEW

The journal lessons are intended to focus more on you, providing practical assessments and the tools you need for your healing journey.

Many of the lessons include: emotional awareness exercises, journaling, identifying thoughts and feelings, determining what you need to feel safe, establishing boundaries, self-care, and more.

Starting in Chapter 4, new tools are introduced to expand your level of awareness and challenge you to make intentional changes that will lead to lasting health. This includes The FASTER Scale and Group Check-In, as well as identifying your personal promises, a Commitment to Change, and using the Double Bind exercise.

The journal lessons work in tandem with the workbook lessons. The combined *Workbook* and *Journal* curriculum was created to provide a holistic approach to healing from betrayal trauma: physically, emotionally, mentally, spiritually, and relationally.

Group Guidelines

The group guidelines should be observed in all Pure Desire groups.

CONFIDENTIALITY

What is said in a group is presented in trust and confidence. It should be given the utmost consideration and privacy and never shared outside the group. Even with spouses, information about another group member's story should not be shared without that person's consent. In order to protect confidentiality, the group is not open to guests or visitors. Anyone who is considering joining the group after it has launched needs to go directly to the group leader.

RESPECT OTHERS

Self-focus, listen respectfully, limit sharing, and respect others

Speak only for yourself, avoid giving advice, and allow others the time to formulate their answers and come to their conclusion. Do not contribute to side conversations and give everyone an opportunity to share.

COMMITMENT TO ACCOUNTABILITY

Regular attendance, take ownership, and be responsible

Make attending group a priority and let your leader or co-leader know if you cannot attend a meeting. Reach out to another group member at least once a week for connection, support, and to share prayer requests. If you feel uncomfortable at any time with something being done in the group, talk with your leader or group.

Group leaders also need to be accountable to the church. It is important for group leaders to submit to the leadership of the church, adhering to all leadership policies and requirements set forth by the church. Leaders should also be meeting with the leadership of the church at least once a quarter to report the successes and challenges groups are seeing.

Pure Desire online group leaders will be accountable to Pure Desire.

COMPLETE HOMEWORK

Complete homework and stay on subject

Homework facilitates the journey to healing. Allow 20-30 minutes each day to complete your homework. Every group member that completes the homework has the opportunity to participate in sharing and making a contribution to the group. The homework needs to be done in writing and includes the assignment for that week. Do your best to stay on topic and minimize drifting off-topic.

MEMO OF UNDERSTANDING
For All Groups

It is important to understand the purpose and parameters of Pure Desire groups and the moral and ethical obligations of group leaders outlined in the Memo of Understanding. This document must be signed before an individual joins the group. Make no exceptions!

Group Structure

Each group session is two hours and accommodates this 40-60-20 plan:

40 MINUTES

The first 40 minutes is a time for women to share their *Journal* responses for the week. This may include various topics such as what they're learning about self-care, safety, and emotional health; recognizing what they're thankful for; identifying how they did on their Commitment to Change and/or where they were on the FASTER Scale. The purpose of this time is to help women become more aware of the healing processes that are at work in their lives.

60 MINUTES

The next 60 minutes is reserved for discussing the workbook lesson and homework assigned for the week. It is important for women to come to group each week with their homework completed. If their homework is not complete, they may not share on the sections that are incomplete. Even if their homework is not completed, women are encouraged to attend group, since so much is gleaned through gathering together and hearing other's share. Never read through the lessons as a group; instead, ask women to highlight information that stood out to them and guide the women through sharing the answers to the questions.

20 MINUTES

Each group ends with a brief look at the next lesson, highlighting any specific areas that may need extra thought or attention, and prayer. This is also time for women to identify their Commitment to Change for the coming week and make arrangements to contact other group members during the week. Connecting during the week helps to create supportive relationships among women who understand the healing process, which moves them away from isolation and into healthy community.

Pure Desire Groups Best Practices

The following practices help ensure a positive, effective group experience and should be observed along with the practices described in the Memo of Understanding (MOU) and Group Guidelines (GG) as communicated in Pure Desire publications.

INCLUDING NEW MEMBERS

- For groups focused on betrayal (*Betrayal & Beyond* for women), we do not recommend adding new members after the group has started. This should only be done with extreme discretion and careful consideration by the leader.
- A new member should join at whatever lesson the group is currently on. We do not recommend attempting to have group members working on different lessons. Progress through the material as a group.

GROUP SIZE

Effective groups will be between four and seven people. We do not recommend starting a group with less than four, as attrition of members up front is common. If the group grows beyond seven members, the group should multiply with a new leader or break into multiple discussion groups for the homework.

MEETING TIME FRAME

The group meeting time is two hours. If the material is covered in less time, the group may break early. When the group reaches two hours, the group should pick up next week where they left off. Committing to end at two hours regardless keeps the group focused and helps avoid rabbit trails.

GROUP LENGTH

Groups should not cover more than one lesson in each meeting, so that group members may fully process the lesson. Some lessons may take more than one week. For Betrayal & Beyond groups, the group will meet for no less than eight months, and may last as long as 12 months.

GROUP PARTICIPATION

Everyone participates in every meeting, unless they haven't completed their homework. Group leaders should facilitate conversation in a way that everyone has time to participate and share. A group member should not be forced to share anything they aren't ready to share yet.

Pure Desire Podcast & Blog

The Pure Desire Podcast and Blog can be an extra source of encouragement throughout your healing journey. Pure Desire releases a new podcast episode weekly and a new blog biweekly. The podcast guests and blog authors consist of Pure Desire staff, individuals and couples who've found healing through Pure Desire, and outside experts within the field of sexual health. The topics discussed include: addiction, betrayal, groups, recovery, healing, emotional health, marriage, sexuality, parenting, resources, tools, and so much more.

 YOU CAN FIND THE PURE DESIRE PODCAST EPISODES AT **PUREDESIRE.ORG/PODCASTS** OR WHEREVER YOU LISTEN TO PODCASTS.

 YOU CAN FIND THE PURE DESIRE BLOG AT **PUREDESIRE.ORG/BLOG**.

Note: If you are feeling triggered by any of the lesson content or this healing process, and want to pursue professional help, please contact Pure Desire at 503-489-0230 or visit **puredesire.org/counseling**.

Memo of Understanding

Pure Desire Group Participants: *Please read and sign this Memo of Understanding, indicating that you have read and understand the purpose and parameters of the Betrayal & Beyond groups and the moral and ethical obligations of leaders.*

I understand that every attempt will be made to guard my anonymity and confidentiality in this group, but that anonymity and confidentiality cannot be absolutely guaranteed in a group setting.

- I realize that the group leader or facilitator cannot control the actions of others in the group.
- I realize that confidentiality is sometimes broken accidentally and without malice.

I understand that the group leader or facilitator is morally and ethically obligated to discuss with me any of the following behaviors, and that this may lead to the breaking of confidentiality and/or possibly intervention:

- I communicate anything that may be interpreted as a threat to self-inflict physical harm.
- I communicate an intention to harm another person.
- I reveal ongoing sexual or physical abuse.
- I exhibit an impaired mental state.

I understand that the Betrayal & Beyond group leader or facilitator may be a mandatory reporter to authorities of sexual conduct that includes minor children, the elderly, or the disabled.

I have been advised that the consequences for communicating the above types of information may include reports to the proper authorities—the police, suicide units or children's protective agencies, as well as to any potential victims.

I understand that this is a Christ-centered group that integrates recovery tools with the Bible and prayer, and that all members may not be of my particular church background. I realize that the Bible may be discussed more (or less) than I would like it to be.

I understand that this is a support group and not a therapy group and that the leader/facilitator is qualified by "life experience" and not by professional training as a therapist or counselor. The leader's or facilitator's role in this group is to create a climate where healing may occur, to support my personal work toward recovery, and to share her own experience, strength, and hope.

Name (please print) _____ Date _____

Signature _____

Witness: Betrayal & Beyond Group Leader's Name _____

Betrayal & Beyond Leader's Signature _____

1

CHAPTER ONE

What Just Happened to Me ?

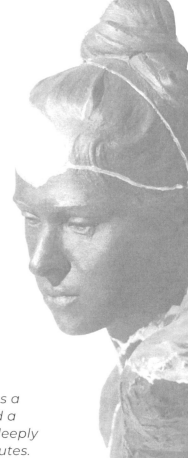

Why Do I Feel So Alone ?

I have been married 25 years and have three children. My husband was a missionary kid who also pastored for 16 years. I always thought we had a good marriage, but now I am wondering if it was all a charade. He is deeply enmeshed in sexual addiction: porn, masturbation, affairs, and prostitutes. He has lived a double life for who knows how long. He says the last few years have been the worst, but admits to having a "full body massage" at a seedy place soon after we were married. He has been out of the ministry for the last few years. I feel manipulated, played, and used. I still love him, but he has become a stranger in many ways. We are currently separated since I found out he is still having an affair with a new girl he met six weeks ago. I need help.

AMY

Like Amy, you have discovered a new reality about your husband. His hidden life has been exposed and you feel alone in your pain, not knowing where to turn for answers or help. Hopefully, the information in this *Workbook* will answer many of your questions, help you process the pain and trauma you're experiencing, and help you recognize that you are not alone.

The following are more stories from women who recently discovered their husband's secret sexual behavior.

My husband accidentally sent me an email meant for an old high school girlfriend. Apparently at their last reunion (which I was unable to attend) they reconnected, and have been sexting ever since. We have been married for almost 12 years and I don't know where to turn.

SUE

Even before we were married, I knew about his struggle with pornography. He said he would try to stop, but that was more than 10 years ago. My husband continues to relapse and confesses it to me when it happens. Each time is a crushing blow. I'm filled with so much pain, shame, and hopelessness. I don't know how much more of this I can take.

CHANTELLE

My husband said he had to do overtime at work. Because a prostitute threatened to contact me if he didn't give her more money, he decided to disclose to me. I was devastated when I realized this has been going on for years. I was also angry at all the sacrifices I made, feeling like a single mom at times, because he was having to work "overtime." Now I have to endure the humiliation of having an STD test. I'm not sure I can go on being married to this man.

CHERYL

My husband was just fired from his job because he was using the work computer for Internet porn. I thought we had the perfect family and he is an elder in our church. I feel there must be something wrong with me that he would risk his job to feed his addiction to porn.

SADIE

Before we were married my husband admitted to struggling with porn and had admitted to a few sexual relationships. But he became a Christian and said that activity was behind him and Christ had healed him. I just discovered he has been on Craigslist looking for women to hook up with. At first, he lied and denied going to those places, then finally admitted he has struggled all 15 years of our marriage. He said he is willing to get help, but I don't know where to go from here.

DENISE

I just found out my husband has had one-night stands at various times during our 18 years of marriage, not just with women, but also with some men. My heart is broken and I don't know if I can continue no matter how much he says he wants help and wants the marriage. Can marriages like mine heal?

APRIL

✚ With whose story can you most identify? Explain.

Aprils story is similar to mine. My husband disclosed that he had a sexical relationship with another guy when he was a teen. This man has stayed with us off and on and David stayed with him and I will always wonder now.

✚ What thoughts and feelings do you have after reading these stories?

I'm angry and sad for them and myself.

Like these women you might have been blindsided by a storm of lies, secrets, and betrayal. You may feel as though you are anchored in the murky waters of despair and grief. So much of what you thought was true about your relationship has turned out to be a lie, and now navigating through life seems impossible.

In the weeks and months ahead, you will be challenged to pull up the anchor that has been immersed in deception, lies, and denial. The journey you are about to embark upon will take you to the deeper clear waters of truth. Venturing out beyond your comfort zone will challenge you to look at what has been an illusion rather than reality. At times, the reality will be difficult but you won't be alone. If you have joined a support group, you will have a group of women who will help you navigate to the crystal clear waters of truth and your anchor will be secure in those new places. As Scripture promises:

> We have this hope as an anchor for the soul, firm and secure. It enters the inner sanctuary behind the curtain, where our forerunner, Jesus, has entered on our behalf.
>
> HEBREWS 6:19-20B (NIV)

Your anchor is only as secure as that to which it is fastened. As you anchor yourself in Christ, He will be the safe harbor for your soul. He understands the betrayal and shame you are facing because He experienced it. Jesus was betrayed by His closest friends and suffered the shame of the cross. Yet, Scripture says He refused the shame (Hebrews 12:2). Throughout your journey, Jesus will show you how to do the same.

The Bible tells us that David also navigated his way through the betrayal of his father-in-law, Saul, who was king over Israel. Saul's scheme was to hunt down and kill David due to jealousy. Hear David's fears as he laments before the Lord in Psalm 55 (NLT):

> *Please listen and answer me, for I am overwhelmed by my troubles. (Verse 2)*
>
> *My heart pounds in my chest. The terror of death assaults me. (Verse 4)*
>
> *Fear and trembling overwhelm me, and I can't stop shaking. (Verse 5)*
>
> *I would fly far away to the quiet of the wilderness. (Verse 7)*
>
> *It is not an enemy who taunts me—I could bear that. It is not my foes who so arrogantly insult me—I could have hidden from them.*
>
> *Instead, it is you—my equal, my companion and close friend. What good fellowship we once enjoyed as we walked together to the house of God. (Verses 12-14)*
>
> *As for my companion, he betrayed his friends; he broke his promises. His words are as smooth as butter, but in his heart is war. His words are as soothing as lotion, but underneath are daggers! (Verses 20-21)*

✝ **How can you relate to what David is feeling?**

I can relate because I am overwhelmed and have a lot of anxiety and the betrayal by someone who is supposed to have your back is awful.

✚ **What promises made to you were broken? What lies have you been told?**

- To love honor and protect, to keep me safe.
That I was safe with him forever and always.
- Nobody else will ever love you, this is your
fault.

David's physical shaking and his desperate desire to flee are both signs of trauma and are natural limbic responses when stress feels overwhelming. The limbic brain, also known as the survival brain, will respond to danger in three ways: fight, flight, or freeze.[1] Like David, you may have some of these same instincts to freeze or be in a state of shock, yet also want to flee and escape perilous circumstances.

These are common symptoms among women who have experienced betrayal trauma. While this list is not exhaustive, it highlights reactions that follow a perceived threat, when our brain responds to trauma with flight and/or freeze behaviors:[2]

- ☑ Helplessness
- ☑ Anxiety
- ☑ Immobility
- ☑ Withdrawing

- ☑ Depression
- ☑ Avoidance
- ☑ Reliving the event
- ☑ Restlessness

- ☑ Denial
- ☑ Confusion
- ☑ Chronic Fatigue
- ☑ Dissociation

✚ **In the above table. check all the symptoms you've experienced. Which of these symptoms have you struggled with the most after** ~~discovery~~ *the abuse.* ~~of your husband's sexually compulsive behavior?~~ **Explain.**

Withdrawing, anxiety, avoidance, depression,
dissociation

[1] H. Stefan Bracha, "Freeze, Flight, Fight, Fright, Faint: Adaptationist Perspectives on the Acute Stress Response Spectrum," *CNS Spectrums 9(9)*, 2004: 679-685.

[2] Barbara Steffens and Marsha Means, *Your Sexually Addicted Spouse: How Partners Can Cope And Heal* (Far Hills: New Horizon Press, 2009), 6-7.

David underlines the fact that the betrayer spoke soothing words and yet his heart was filled with deceit. You, too, may have been caught up in the smooth talking and deceptive behavior of a betrayer, all of which now turns out to be a pile of lies. At this point, there have been so many lies you might not know what to believe. Even if there has been some discovery or disclosure, you may still question, "What is a lie and what is truth?"

From David's experience we can draw out a powerful truth. The only way to pull the anchor out of the murky waters of deceit and lies is to begin to **believe the behavior and not the words.** Those caught up in out-of-control sexual behavior are masters of manipulation and deception because they have had to keep the duplicity of their lives hidden. Even if they have a commitment to Christ, they have literally compartmentalized their lives so they can carry on two lives at once—a public life and a private life. This double life probably began at an early age. They brought these behaviors into the marriage relationship, which is key to understanding that their addiction is not your fault. Living together in marriage has required a new level of charm and deceit on the addict's part to cover his lies and addictive behavior.

Paul warns that when Christians are unable to surrender the darkness of their addiction to Christ's healing light, they will develop a hard heart.

> *So I tell you this, and insist on it in the Lord, that you must no longer live as the Gentiles do, in the futility of their thinking. They are darkened in their understanding and separated from the life of God because of the ignorance that is in them due to the hardening of their hearts. Having lost all sensitivity, they have given themselves over to sensuality so as to indulge in every kind of impurity, and they are full of greed.*
>
> EPHESIANS 4:17-19 (NIV)

This continual openness to sensuality allows darkness to control their minds. The progression leads to a callous heart, to a deadened spirit and, finally, to a fully addicted heart. Deception is so integrated into their lives that denial becomes a primary coping strategy, even when unnecessary. It usually takes a crisis—such as being found out, the possibility of facing criminal charges, or the possibility of losing their marriage—to wake them up to their desperate need for radical help.

✚ **How have you seen a calloused heart toward you and the Lord developing in your spouse? Explain.**

He stopped going to church with us and he was ~~never~~ always sorry at first but then over time he stopped apologizing and blamed ~~the~~ me.

✚ **How did you discover the betrayal?**

He disclosed the sexual nature with the man and he abused me.

✚ **What were your initial thoughts? Feelings? Behaviors?**

to shut down, I thought it was better that we have an intact family than a broken one.

In conclusion, let's consider again David's words in Psalm 55:15 (NLT):

> Let death stalk my enemies; let the grave swallow them alive, for evil makes its home within them.

✚ On a scale of 1-10 (10 being extremely angry), how angry are you about the betrayal you have experienced? Circle the appropriate corresponding number.

1	2	3	4	5	6	7	8	9	10

Not angry   Angry   Extremely Angry

✚ Explain your score.

I'm as angry as I can be Because I'm still in the middle of it and he continues to betray me and the boys.

It is normal for you to be outraged at the intense betrayal, deception, and manipulation that has been used against you for selfish, addictive purposes. You may even feel entirely numb toward your spouse without feeling any loving emotions. Considering the trauma you have experienced, both responses are natural ways for your soul to try to protect itself from his hurtful actions.

But there is hope, no matter how numb and angry you are. Hope begins when you make a choice to pull up your anchor out of the murky waters of deception and move into a new place of reality in which **you believe his behaviors and not his words.**

✚ What hope do you have in light of what you have learned from this lesson and reading God's Word?

I have alot of hope that things will get better.

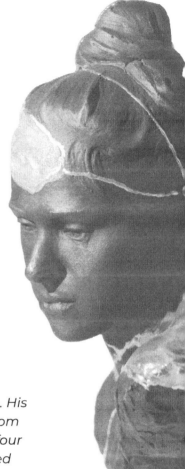

Why It's Not My Fault

My husband recently shared with me his past that had been well hidden. His family had many dark secrets and to this day he struggles with things from his past. My husband's earliest memories of sexual abuse began at age four at the hands of his older sister and then his older brother. He remembered pornography in the house. This activity continued into young adulthood. Masturbation started at a young age and has continued throughout his adulthood. He remembers his father talking to the boys inappropriately about sex and how they would never measure up to how good he was with the ladies. My husband admits that he is most vulnerable to this addiction when he is experiencing high stress. But he wants to be free of this bondage. My heart was broken when all this was brought to light. Is there any hope for healing?

BETH

At this point, it may feel hopeless. Because of what you've experienced, it may be difficult to trust God or trust that life will ever get back to normal again. And while some things have changed forever because of the betrayal, there is hope in the possibility of creating something better for you and your future.

> *Be strong and take heart, all you who hope in the Lord.*
> PSALM 31:24 (NIV)

There is hope, although you may not feel it now. God loves you so much and His heart breaks over what you've experienced through betrayal. He wants the very best for you and will work with you to heal your heart and restore you to a place of health and wholeness.

✚ **If you had one hope for healing at this point, what would it be? Explain.**

_____

_____

_____

_____

_____

_____

As mentioned in the previous lesson, because of the addict's lies and manipulative behavior, reality has been hard to grasp. But what does this mean?

Note: _We are using the term "addict" and/or "addiction" to describe hidden, compulsive, or problematic sexual behaviors in general. We are not assessing your loved one to be "addicted" but rather are describing a pattern of behavior over time._

To get a better understanding of what you've experienced, here are a few definitions to help explain some of an addict's behaviors:

- **Lie:** an intentionally false statement; present a false impression, be deceptive.
- **Manipulate:** alter or present so as to mislead.
- **Deceive:** cause someone to believe something that is not true, typically in order to gain some personal advantage.
- **Gaslight:** manipulate someone by psychological means into questioning their own sanity.

You have been lied to. You have been manipulated. You have been deceived. You have been put in situations that caused you to question your reality. None of this is your fault.

✚ **What thoughts and feelings do you have about learning these definitions?**

_____

_____

_____

_____

_____

_____

_____

✝ **Have you experienced any of these behaviors ? Give one example that comes to mind.**

_____

_____

_____

_____

_____

_____

_____

_____

_____

_____

_____

This week we are moving out of the murky waters of deception and into the deep waters of reality where we will be anchored for many weeks. Raising awareness of what you've experienced, and recognizing when these behaviors are being used against you, will empower you to keep moving forward on this journey.

One of the first realities to address is the fact that your husband's addiction is not your fault. As you can see from Beth's heartbreaking story, her husband's sexual issues began many years before they met, which is likely the case with your spouse. Also, there seems to be a generational element with the father's attitude and the siblings' involvement. God tells us about generational curses in Deuteronomy:

> _For I, the Lord your God, am a jealous God, visiting the iniquity of the fathers upon the children to the third and fourth generations of those who hate Me, but showing mercy to thousands, to those who love Me and keep My commandments._
>
> DEUTERONOMY 5:9B-10 (NKJV)

When we pursue healing, it breaks any generational curses that may be impacting us and allows God's blessings to flow through our lives to the thousandth generation.

✚ With what you know about your husband's struggles, have you observed any generational elements that could be contributing to his behaviors? Explain.

_____

_____

_____

_____

_____

_____

_____

_____

_____

Your husband's sexual addiction is never your fault. This was likely his struggle years before he met you. He brought this into the relationship. **All of his choices and his behaviors are on him.**

And while this is 100% true, his behaviors have impacted you. His behaviors have hurt you. Raising awareness of how you've been impacted is important for your healing.

How has the addict's behavior affected you?

✚ Check the behaviors you have experienced:

☐ The addict blamed me for his unmet needs.

☐ I've experienced a lack of emotional intimacy and/or connectedness.

☐ I've experienced shame and humiliation because of his sexual activity.

☐ I've suffered financial losses.

☐ I've been exposed to the physical risk of HIV and/or STIs/STDs (sexually transmitted infections/diseases).

☐ When I've brought up a problem, it somehow becomes my problem.

☐ _____

☐ _____

☐ _____

If any or all of these factors are true, your relationship has been suffering for years. Your husband has spent a lot of time in the relationship trying to convince you that what "was true" was only imaginary. You may have spent a lot of time trying to prove that he was not telling the truth. And now that many of his behaviors have come to light, you can see the various ways it has impacted your relationship.

✚ **When did you begin to notice your relationship was suffering? Explain.**

_____

_____

_____

_____

_____

_____

_____

_____

✚ **What were the signs?**

_____

_____

_____

_____

_____

_____

_____

_____

Depending on your season of life, healing from betrayal trauma will impact you and may impact others in the family. This is true even if you're engaged and not yet married. Healing and recovery (if you choose to stay in the relationship) may include these three parts:

- Healing for the partner from her betrayal.
- Recovery for the addict from his addition.
- Recovery and healing for the relationship (which may or may not include children too).

These aspects of the healing and recovery process are important for the survival of the relationship.

But right now, your healing is paramount! You are not responsible for anyone else's healing (or recovery), only your own. You have to focus on what you need to find healing from betrayal and God wants to meet you exactly where you are. Although many areas of your life may feel uncertain at this point, take time to rest in God's love and protection over you.

✚ Write out Psalm 91 in your own handwriting and replace "Whoever" with "I will..."

Whoever dwells in the shelter of the Most High will rest in the shadow of the Almighty. I will say of the Lord, "He is my refuge and my fortress, my God, in whom I trust."

PSALM 91:1-2 (NIV)

HOW CAN GOD BE YOUR FORTRESS THIS WEEK?

✝ **Fill in the blanks with either "I," "my," or "me" or your name and then read it out loud to yourself.**

He shall cover _____ with His feathers, And under His wings _____ shall take refuge; His truth shall be _____ shield and buckler. _____ shall not be afraid of the terror by night, Nor of the arrow that flies by day, Nor of the pestilence that walks in darkness, Nor of the destruction that lays waste at noonday.

PSALM 91:4-6 (NKJV)

For he will command his angels concerning _____ to guard _____ in all [my] ways; they will lift _____ up in their hands, so that _____ will not strike [my] foot against a stone. _____ will tread on the lion and the cobra; _____ will trample the great lion and the serpent. "Because [she] loves me," says the Lord, "I will rescue [her]; I will protect [her], for [she] acknowledges my name. _____ will call on me, and I will answer [her]; I will be with _____ in trouble...

PSALM 91:11-15A (NIV)

✝ **After reading this modified version out loud to yourself, describe any thoughts and feelings you have about these Scriptures.**

_____

_____

_____

_____

_____

_____

_____

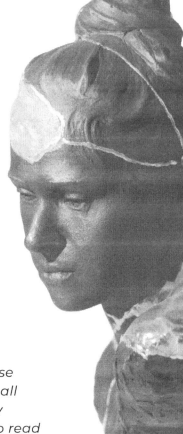

What Do I Do Now ?

I just got a copy of the book "Pure Desire" and started reading it because I was desperate. I realize my dad, and now the men I have dated, have all struggled with this issue. I was ready to call off my relationship with my current boyfriend because of this issue in his life. I gave him the book to read and I cannot believe the transformation. He wants to come back to church and really wants to pursue our relationship in a healthy way. I read your chapter in the book and realized the part about having two different realities describes us and our relationship. It was also disappointing to realize it could take up to five years for real healing to come. I don't know what to do.

DONNA

Donna is not alone. She and many other women, married and single, have realized their husband (or boyfriend in this case) has a different reality when disclosure (or discovery) happens.

Donna is referring to the following information that delineates the difference in "His Reality" and "Her Reality" after disclosure:[3]

---

[3] Scot Oja, For Men Only 90 Day Covenant as referenced in *Betrayed Heart for Women Only* (Gresham: East Hill Church, 2004), 45.

HIS REALITY

- ☐ I'm becoming a man of integrity.
- ☐ I've never loved her more.
- ☐ I'm beginning to see how much I value our marriage.
- ☐ Finally, I'm an honest man.
- ☐ I understand the healing process sometimes takes three to five years. I'm sure I can complete this process in a couple of years.

HER REALITY

- ☐ I've been betrayed.
- ☐ I've never felt less loved or worthy.
- ☐ I've never realized until now how little the marriage meant to him.
- ☐ How could he live a lie like this?
- ☐ Five years seems like a lifetime to deal with this pain.

✚ On the above chart, place a check mark next to the statements under "Her Reality" with which you can identify. Under "His Reality," mark with an X the statements you have heard your husband say or reflect his attitudes at this point.

✚ What thoughts and feelings do you have after learning about His Reality and Her Reality? Explain.

_____

_____

_____

_____

_____

_____

These realities bring pain to both the addict and the partner who has been betrayed. The addict has kept his secret life hidden for possibly 20-30 years or more. It has produced a burden of shame and a life of lies. Now for the first time, he is finally allowing the light of Christ to come into those dark areas and the shame is beginning to disappear. In being honest, he is feeling great relief. Think of it this way: for years he has kept his secret life hidden in a dump truck full of dirt, garbage, and other debris (his hidden sexual behaviors). And now, he feels free enough to dump "the truth" on his wife (or girlfriend in this case). She is left buried under a mountain of betrayal, lies, deceit, manipulation, anger, despair, worthlessness, shame, and more.

He feels so good that there are no more secrets and wants her to immediately forgive, so they can "feel okay with each other." He forgets how long he has endured under the burden and struggle of this issue; and how this revelation will devastate her. **She will now have to spend some time sorting out and processing the new reality and how it has impacted her.** Her pain is enormous and she is wondering, "How can I endure this for three to five years?"

You may be in this same place. You might be wondering, *"What do I do now?"* In the following lessons, we will go deeper, helping you process the pain and walk through healing from betrayal.

The journey begins by first identifying what has been dumped on you due to discovery (or disclosure). This may include some of your husband's specific behaviors, which you're now aware of, as well as thoughts and feelings you're now experiencing because of this new awareness. Do your best to identify what you're feeling; if you push down these feelings and suppress them, they may pop up at unexpected times or contribute to feelings of numbness and depression.

WHAT HAS BEEN DUMPED ON YOU?

✚ In the space below, write what you think has been dumped on you: the aspects of your husband's secret life that you now feel buried under?

Examples: *lies, deceit, manipulation, his pornography addiction, emotional affairs with other women, money spent on his addiction, his behaviors when on work trips.*

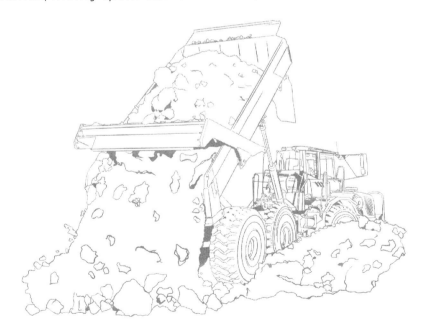

✚ What are your thoughts and feelings about all that has been dumped on you because of his secret life?

Examples: *fear of abandonment, anger over your husband's lies, anger at God, betrayal, shame, financial loss, devaluation, worthlessness, humiliation, confusion, despair.*

_____

_____

_____

_____

_____

_____

_____

_____

As you have identified thoughts and feelings associated with what has been dumped on you, know that real healing comes as you join with other women who can help you dig out from under the mess and begin to process the pain. Fortunately, Donna was in a city where there was a group of women who were ready and eager to help her process this pain. Scripture points out that some burdens are too heavy to carry alone.

> *Carry each other's burdens, and in this way you will fulfill the law of Christ*
> GALATIANS 6:2 (NIV)

In another part of her email, Donna raised the question about forgiveness. This comes up all the time and, again, focuses on the two different realities. The addict assumes since all is out in the open, forgiveness should happen immediately. **In a later chapter, we will spend a number of weeks understanding real forgiveness.** But if forgiveness is given prematurely—given too soon, in an effort to preserve the relationship and before you have processed your anger and grief—you will have to act like nothing's wrong on the outside, but on the inside your heart will be bleeding. **Forgiving too soon will give the addict an illusion of closeness, when in reality, there will be huge pockets of pain in your heart that have not been resolved or healed.**

 Forgiveness should never get ahead of healing trauma.[4]

---

[4] Adrian Hickman, "PSAP, Module 1, Day 2" (presentation, International Institute for Trauma and Addiction Professionals (IITAP), virtual, May 11, 2021).

While forgiveness is a crucial part of the healing journey, partners need to be given time and space to go through the process of forgiving. This is not something that should be done out of obligation, but through intense prayer and the work of the Holy Spirit. It is through this healing process that God transforms and moves a partner's heart to forgiveness.

Addicts are notorious for wanting what they want immediately: in the counseling office, I have told many that they will need to learn to live without forgiveness for a time. **Their wife cannot sacrifice her integrity and safety to satisfy his need for immediate forgiveness.** If a partner gives in too soon, it will only silence her anguish and indignation that will continue to rise to the surface until her heart is healed. Remember, **forgiving too soon only deepens the denial process for both spouses and keeps real change from happening.**

A partner cannot forgive what she doesn't know or understand. The healing and recovery process takes time. We have seen this time and again through staggered disclosures: bits and pieces of the story continuing to come out over time. This tends to retraumatize the partner and she will spend several weeks attempting to understand what she is forgiving.

Choosing to work through the healing process, knowing that it will take time to rebuild trust and safety, is key to reconciliation and creating a new normal. Choosing to surrender to God, and forgive, does not mean we have to trust someone or allow them to continue hurting us. We are choosing to allow God to work and begin this process, understanding that it may include "two steps forward and one step back" as new information is revealed.

✛ With regard to forgiving too soon and the healing process, what thoughts and feelings come to mind after reading this information?

At this point, many betrayed partners feel like their world has been turned upside down. They feel paralyzed and unable to move forward. One study revealed, approximately 72% of women who experienced betrayal suffered "significant distress and impairment in social, occupational, or other important areas of functioning."[5] This disruption to their lives throws off everything: they cannot sleep; they cannot eat; they cannot concentrate. Their mind is consumed by the discovery of their spouse's behaviors and what else they don't know. They withdraw from normal activities. They feel isolated and alone. They are unsure of what the future holds.

The partner of a sex addict has responses that serve as reactions to a stressor that is traumatic in nature, in predictable emotional, behavioral, and physiological ways. She seeks what she cannot find: safety in an unsafe situation.[6]

Right now, your need for safety is normal. The life you had before betrayal probably felt safe in many ways, which turned out to be a false reality. So creating a new definition of safety and what that will look like for you going forward will take time. In the coming weeks, we will work to redefine and reestablish safety, which will be a foundational aspect of your healing.

✚ **Based on your current situation, identify one area of your life in which you would like to focus on redefining and reestablishing safety.**

Examples: *voicing your concerns rather than staying silent; walking away if things get too heated; sleeping in separate rooms until you feel safe; asking him to move out if his angry outbursts continue.*

_____

_____

_____

_____

_____

_____

_____

[5] Barbara A. Steffens & Robyn L. Rennie (2006) The Traumatic Nature of Disclosure for Wives of Sexual Addicts, *Sexual Addiction & Compulsivity*, 13:2-3, 247-267, DOI: 10.1080/10720160600870802.

[6] Barbara Steffens quote, APSATS founding President, apsats.org.

✚ Wherever you're at on this journey—emotionally, mentally, and spiritually—write out a prayer for yourself.

_____

_____

_____

_____

_____

_____

_____

_____

_____

_____

_____

_____

_____

_____

_____

_____

_____

_____

_____

_____

Pray that God will give you the strength and wisdom needed to make wise decisions. Pray He will cover you with the peace and comfort that only His love can bring. Pray that, even in the midst of this difficult season, God will meet you exactly where you're at as you begin to heal your heart and mind from the pain of betrayal.

Note: If you are feeling triggered by any of the lesson content or this healing process, and want to pursue professional help, please contact Pure Desire at 503-489-0230 or visit **puredesire.org/counseling**.

2

Why Do I Feel and Behave the Way I Do ?

What Is Trauma ?

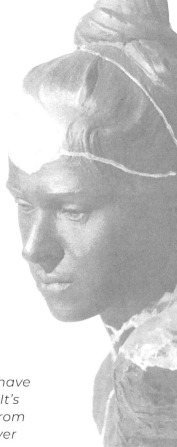

I discovered my husband's pornography addiction three months ago. I have no words to explain the devastation I feel. I'm not even sure what I feel. It's like a switch has flipped in my brain; my every thought destroying me from the inside out. Not only do I replay the moment of discovery over and over in my mind, but every interaction and conversation we've had since. He says it was a one-time thing and doesn't want to talk about it, but I'm not sure I believe him. And I don't feel like I can trust him.

Three months ago, I was happy, energetic, and full of life. And now, I don't know what I am. It's as though all the energy and life has been sucked out of my body and my organs, especially my heart, are struggling to survive.

JAYLA

Dr. Patrick Carnes gives a helpful definition that underlines this truth about the power of betrayal and how traumatic it can be:

> *Betrayal is a breach of trust. What you thought was true—counted on to be true—was not. It was just smoke and mirrors, outright deceit and lies. It was exploitation. You were used...Betrayal is a form of abandonment. Abandonment causes deep shame. Abandonment by betrayal is worse than mindless neglect. Betrayal is purposed and self-serving...If severe enough, it is traumatic.[1]*

---

[1] Patrick Carnes, *The Betrayal Bond: Breaking Free of Exploitive Relationships* (Deerfield Beach: Health Communications, Inc., 1997), xv, xvi.

Understanding the complexity of trauma and its effect on us is not an easy task. Even more so when attempting to grasp the impact of betrayal trauma. To gain a greater understanding of trauma, we'll look at myths surrounding trauma, definitions of trauma, the unique aspects of betrayal trauma, and different types of trauma.

FOUR MYTHS ABOUT TRAUMA:

✚ **Circle any of these four myths you believed about trauma:**

Myth #1: Traumatic experiences are uncommon.

Truth: *The Canadian Journal of Psychiatry* reports over 70% of the adult population experience trauma at some point in their lives.[2]

Myth #2: If people were just stronger, they could get over trauma.

Truth: Responses to trauma vary depending on several factors, such as: the severity of the trauma, an individual's ability to cope with stress, support received following a traumatic experience, previous traumatic experiences, and more.[3]

Myth #3: The only people who have trauma are those who experienced high levels of danger, fear, pain, abuse, or horror; such as sexual assault, a serious car accident, war combat, fire, or natural disasters.

Truth: Trauma can develop from **Big T** experiences (meaning high intensity) and it can also be produced by **little t** experiences (meaning frequency).[4] We will discuss these types of trauma in this lesson.

Myth #4: Those raised in a good Christian home don't usually experience trauma.

Truth: Christians are not exempt from trauma. But as Christians, we have a loving heavenly Father who will help us through the healing process.

---

[2] Naomi Breslau, "Epidemiologic studies of trauma, posttraumatic stress disorder, and other psychiatric disorders," *Canadian Journal of Psychiatry* 2002 Dec; 47(10): 923-929.

[3] Rebecca Bradley and Diane Roberts, *Behind the Mask* (Gresham: Pure Desire Ministries International, 2012), 73-74.

[4] Francine Shapiro, *Eye Movement Desensitization and Reprocessing (EMDR) Therapy: Basic Principles, Protocols, and Procedures*, Third Edition (New York: The Guilford Press, 2018), 4.

"I have told you these things, so that in me you may have peace. In this world you will have trouble. But take heart! I have overcome the world."

JOHN 16:33 (NIV)

✚ **Which of these myths has been most detrimental to you regarding your trauma from betrayal? Explain.**

_____

_____

_____

_____

_____

Trauma is...

When you hear the word "trauma" what comes to mind? Do you think of devastating natural disasters, like hurricanes that level a city, leaving many dead and unaccounted for? Perhaps you think of the thousands of stories of children who have survived various forms of abuse throughout their childhood? Maybe you think of all those who have lived through times of war and civil unrest? Or do you think of the children who come home from school every day to an empty house, whose parents are hard at work, but the child feels neglected and alone?

These are exactly the types of situations and life events that create trauma; the things that happen to us and around us which leave deep wounds in our soul. As we seek to understand and explain how trauma has impacted our lives, the purpose is never to blame anyone. The purpose is to raise awareness to areas of our lives where we carry trauma, so we can begin to heal.

Research commissioned by American Bible Society and conducted by Barna Group presented this narrow definition of trauma:

...physical, psychological or emotional trauma, such as extreme violence, abuse or a near-death experience that produces a response of intense fear, helplessness or horror lasting more than a few weeks.[5]

---

[5] American Bible Society, Trauma in America: *Understanding How People Face Hardships and How the Church Offers Hope* (Ventura: Barna Group, 2020), 13.

Even with this narrow definition, their study revealed that one in five U.S. adults experienced the effects of trauma in the past 10 years. Of the 21 types of traumatic experiences listed in this study, the most common cause of trauma was the death of a loved one. **The second most common cause of trauma was "betrayal by someone you trusted."[6]**

In his book, *The Body Keeps the Score*, Dr. Bessel van der Kolk describes trauma this way:

...trauma produces actual physiological changes, including a recalibration of the brain's alarm system, an increase in stress hormone activity, and alterations in the system that filters relevant information from irrelevant. We now know that trauma compromises the brain area that communicates the physical, embodied feeling of being alive. These changes explain why traumatized individuals become hypervigilant to threat at the expense of spontaneously engaging in their day-to-day lives. They also help us understand why traumatized people so often keep repeating the same problems and have such trouble learning from experience. We now know that their behaviors are not the result of moral failings or signs of lack of willpower or bad character—they are caused by actual changes in the brain.[7]

When talking about trauma, it's important to recognize that the trauma is not the situation or event; the situation or event was traumatic. **The trauma is what we're left with—the residual feelings created that we carry—when the situation or event is over.** Trauma can have a paralyzing effect, keeping us from moving forward. Consider this definition of trauma:

 Trauma overwhelms our capacity to deal with the event in the moment.[8]

We feel distracted and consumed by what we're experiencing. The inciting event has created chaos in our mind and body, completely disrupting our ability to live our life the way we did before our world was turned upside down by betrayal. So when it comes to understanding the effects of trauma, it's not about asking, "What's wrong with me?" It's about asking, "What happened to me?" and working to figure out the answer.

---

[6] American Bible Society, *Trauma in America*, 25.

[7] Bessel van der Kolk, *The Body Keeps the Score: Brain, Mind, and Body in the Healing of Trauma* (New York: Penguin Books, 2014), 2-3.

[8] Craig Cashwell, "PSAP Training Program, Module 2, Day 1," International Institute for Trauma & Addiction Professionals (IITAP), Portland, Oregon, November 1, 2021.

BETRAYAL TRAUMA

There is a uniqueness to betrayal trauma, in that the nature of the relationship contributes to the level of trauma experienced by the partner.[9] Betrayal trauma is compounded by the following elements:[10]

- The violation is done by someone who you depend on for survival, safety, and security.
- The expectation of trust and well-being is significantly violated.
- Results in being less aware or unable to recall the traumatic experience; doing so would threaten the relationship and individual's survival.

For some women who experience betrayal, this can lead to Post-Traumatic Stress Disorder (PTSD): experiencing extreme distress and disruption to their daily lives, which resulted from a traumatic event.[11] Symptoms include:

- Intrusive thoughts and memories of the traumatic event.
- Avoidance of thoughts and behaviors that bring up memories of the event: people, places, activities, specific situations.
- Negative changes in thoughts and mood: isolated and withdrawn; increased negative view of self and others; uninterested in previously enjoyed activities; lack of positive emotions.
- Changes in arousal and reactivity: difficulty concentrating; heightened startle response or on high alert; increased aggressive response; sleep disturbances.

When struggling with PTSD, many women will exhibit several of the above symptoms for one month or more, which completely disrupts all areas of their life.

Even more so, the trauma some partners experience is best defined as Complex PTSD.

Complex PTSD is typically the result of exposure to repeated or prolonged instances or multiple forms of interpersonal trauma, often occurring under circumstances where escape is not possible due to physical, psychological, maturational, family/ environmental, or social constraints.[12]

---

[9] Barbara Steffens, "APSATS MPTM 4 Day Training," The Association of Partners of Sex Addicts Trauma Specialists, Online, Day 1, June 11, 2021

[10] Gilbert Reyes, Jon Elhai, and Julian Ford, *The Encyclopedia of Psychological Trauma* (Hoboken: John Wiley & Sons, Inc, 2008), 76.

[11] Matthew Tull, "What Is Post-Traumatic Stress Disorder?" *Verywell Mind*, October 27, 2021, https://www.verywellmind.com/ptsd-in-the-dsm-5-2797324.

[12] Barbara Steffens, "APSATS MPTM 4 Day Training," The Association of Partners of Sex Addicts Trauma Specialists, Online, Day 1, June 11, 2021.

Through betrayal, many partners have survived repeated traumatic experiences—years of lies, deception, and manipulation—without actually recognizing the extent of how it's impacting their mind, body, and soul.

✚ **As you read through this section about the various forms of trauma, which symptoms are affecting you most due to betrayal?**

_____

_____

_____

_____

✚ **When learning that trauma is not the event itself but the residual feelings created by the event, what feelings can you identify that you carry on a regular basis since discovery (or disclosure)?**

_____

_____

_____

_____

_____

We looked at several myths surrounding trauma. Let's now look at three truths about trauma.

Truth One: The way we experience trauma is unique to us.

God created each of us as unique human beings. He gave each of us a specific temperament and personality that make us distinct. Our God-given characteristics and qualities shape who we are and how we process our world. And all of these things will influence how we experience trauma.

For example, upon discovery of her husband's hidden sexual behaviors, a partner may become angry, immediately confront her husband, and want to know everything. Or she might become angry, pack a bag, and leave. Or perhaps she cries and seeks a place of solitude, replaying the scene over and over in her head. Or maybe she is in shock and disbelief, she's devastated; yet reaches out to a friend for comfort and counsel before making any decisions. Or a million other possible responses to the trauma created through discovery.

All of these responses are normal and will likely be very different for each partner.

This is also true for the women in this group. There may be women who have a similar story, yet the impact of the trauma may be more severe for one than the other. We each have different life experiences, so we cannot compare our trauma or our responses to anyone else—even though there may be similarities in our stories. For this reason, it's important to not compare trauma.

The only thing we can compare are the enemy's lies–they are always the same:

- You are not enough.
- There is something wrong with you.
- You are the only one who feels this way.
- You will never measure up to his fantasies.
- You are the problem in the marriage.
- If you would just give him more sex, this wouldn't have happened.

All trauma is significant and the way we experience trauma is unique to each of us.

Because of this, our healing journey will also have elements that are specific to our situation and may take longer to process. This is okay.

What is most important is that you keep moving forward with healing the trauma you've experienced through betrayal.

✚ **What aspects of your situation are unique or different from others you've heard?**

_____

_____

_____

_____

_____

_____

✝ **What characteristics and qualities has God given you that will equip and strengthen you on this healing journey ?**

_____

_____

_____

_____

_____

_____

Truth Two: Trauma can render us emotionally speechless.

Trauma, by its very nature, has a tendency to leave us speechless. Not only because we are physiologically unable to put our feelings into words, but more so because we've never felt this way before and cannot articulate what it is we're actually feeling.

A Chinese proverb describes this dilemma: _"The deepest pain has no words."_

Whether we realize it or not, trauma reverberates throughout our brain and body in a unique way, creating chaos within several systems. For example, when we experience trauma, our brain produces neurochemical reactions that deactivate Broca's area of the brain.[13] This is significant because Broca's area is the part of our brain that translates our feelings into words. One author describes it this way:

 Feeling helpless against a dire threat, people may experience numbness, withdrawal, confusion, shock, or speechless terror.[14]

...traumatized people often have enormous difficulty telling other people what has happened to them. Their bodies reexperiences terror, rage, and helplessness, as well as the impulse to fight or flee, but these feelings are almost impossible to articulate. Trauma by nature drives us to the edge of comprehension, cutting us off from language based on common experience or an imaginable past.[15]

---

[13] Carol Juergensen Sheets, "APSATS MPTM 4 Day Training," The Association of Partners of Sex Addicts Trauma Specialists, Online, Day 2, June 12, 2021.

[14] Bessel van der Kolk, "In Terror's Grip: Healing the Ravages of Trauma," _Cerebrum_, 4, January 2002.

[15] Bessel van der Kolk, _The Body Keeps the Score: Brain, Mind, and Body in the Healing of Trauma_ (New York: Penguin Books, 2014), 43.

As a betrayed partner, when considering all we have been through and are continuing to heal from, it makes sense that we would struggle to find the words to say in the moment.

Being part of this group, taking the time to discover how trauma is impacting your life, and giving yourself grace throughout this process are some of the best things you can do for yourself. It's okay to take it slow. Be intentional. Exploring your feelings and being able to put words to your feelings, and communicate your feelings in a healthy way, will give you a strong foundation for moving forward in your healing.

✚ **When have you found it difficult to put your feelings into words? Explain.**

_____

_____

_____

_____

_____

_____

_____

_____

_____

_____

_____

_____

Truth Three: Trauma comes in many forms.

Trauma comes in many forms but we're going to focus on two extremes of trauma: **Big T** trauma (events of extreme impact) and **little t** trauma (small events that occur over and over again).[16] On the surface, little t traumatic events (trauma of abandonment) may appear to be totally insignificant, but their cumulative effect can be as devastating as a single massive Big T traumatic event (trauma of infringement). Both types of trauma can lead to high levels of internal pain and can trigger a myriad of responses.

---

[16] Francine Shapiro, _Eye Movement Desensitization and Reprocessing (EMDR) Therapy: Basic Principles, Protocols, and Procedures_, Third Edition (New York: The Guilford Press, 2018), 4.

TYPES OF TRAUMA GRAPH[17]

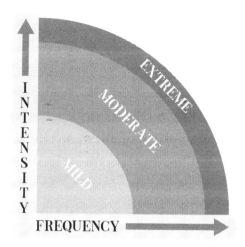

Trauma of Infringement

- Combat experiences
- Rape
- Sexual abuse
- Punching
- Slapping
- Verbal attacks
- Demeaning nicknames

Trauma of Abandonment

- Silence
- Neglect
- Lack of support
- Open rejection

Trauma of infringement reflects things done to us and are characterized by the intensity of the event. This typically includes experiences of high intensity, such as combat, natural disaster, rape or sexual assault, extreme physical or verbal abuse, and more. In many cases, this type of traumatic event is infrequent, but intense.

Trauma of abandonment reflects things kept from us and are characterized by the frequency of the event. This typically includes experiences of neglect, a lack of support, open rejection, and more. In many cases, this type of traumatic event happens over and over, even consistently, but is more mild, comparatively.

Naturally, we might think that infringement trauma would have a greater impact; however, as indicated on the above graph, abandonment trauma can be equally devastating and profoundly impact our lives.

For example, the discovery of your husband's compulsive sexual behaviors is a high intensity event and can result in extreme trauma. However, if your husband continues to lie about his porn use, this may not be as intense, but may happen with greater frequency. This can result in extreme trauma.

An important step in healing trauma happens through recognizing and acknowledging big and little traumatic experiences. So let's look at the various experiences you've had since discovery (or disclosure). In each category of trauma, infringement and abandonment, add examples from your experiences in the space provided. Keep in mind: each person may categorize intensity/frequency within the context of their own experiences.[18] Some examples are given to get you started.

---

[17] Ted Roberts, *Seven Pillars of Freedom Workbook* (Gresham: Pure Desire Ministries International, 2015), 161.

[18] Rebecca Bradley and Diane Roberts, *Behind the Mask* (Gresham: Pure Desire Ministries International, 2012), 76-77.

✚ In the table below, list your trauma of infringement (high intensity: things done to you):

High Intensity

Examples: *Discovery of my husband's affair; My husband lost his job for looking at porn at work; Discovered how much money my husband has spent on his acting out behaviors throughout our marriage...*

Medium Intensity

Examples: *My husband has commented about other women when we're together; My husband has lied about the extent of his porn use...*

Low Intensity

Example: *My husband has criticized how I look/dress...*

Now let's consider the trauma of abandonment or smaller experiences that may have occurred over and over again. Remember, negative frequent events can cause an accumulation of pain, as seen at the bottom of the Types of Trauma graph. As Dr. Patrick Carnes points out, "Little acts of degradation, manipulation, secrecy, and shame on a daily basis take their toll. Trauma by accumulation sneaks up on its victims."[19]

---

[19] Patrick Carnes, *The Betrayal Bond: Breaking Free of Exploitive Relationships* (Deerfield Beach: Health Communications, Inc., 1997), 5.

✚ On the table below, list your trauma of abandonment (high frequency: things kept from you):

High Intensity

Example: *My husband uses porn/masturbation on a regular basis instead of having sex with me...*

Medium Intensity

Examples: *My husband continually lies about where he is and what he's doing; My husband blames me for his porn use...*

Low Intensity

Example: *My husband continually puts work before spending time with me...*

✚ After filling out your trauma of infringement and trauma of abandonment chart, think about what messages were communicated to you through these experiences. What messages do you carry as a result of these experiences?

_____

_____

_____

_____

_____

_____

Trauma's Influence in My Healing Journey

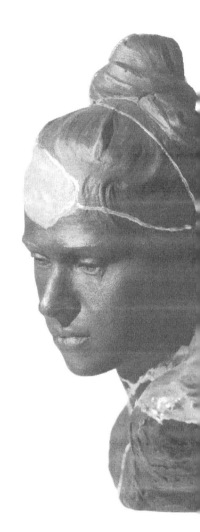

I don't know what's happening to me. I can't stop crying, which is confusing and scaring my kids. I'm filled with anxiety and cannot seem to talk myself off the ledge. My mind is spinning; consumed by what I found on the computer and overwhelmed by the thought of what my husband has been doing. I feel afraid, but afraid of what? I can't eat. Or sleep. I'm constantly on edge. I'm unable to shake the feeling that something bad is about to happen.

JORDYN

For many betrayed partners, the trauma we experience can have a powerful and long-lasting effect in our lives, especially if left untreated. In their book, *Your Sexually Addicted Spouse*, the authors equate the effects of a husband's sexual addiction to that of an earthquake.

If one lives through a terrible earthquake, he or she will feel terrified when the ground shakes again, even if it is only a minor tremor. Just as living through a bad earthquake produces trauma, so, too, does living through the discovery that one's partner is a sex addict. Sex addiction produces a life-quake, leaving traumatic effects on a relationship and on lives. When new tremors—or even perceived tremors—occur, an already traumatized partner almost always has a stress response, just like an earthquake survivor does.[20]

✚ **How does this earthquake analogy resonate with you?**

_____

_____

_____

_____

_____

_____

_____

_____

Most of the time, our response to trauma is a means to protect ourselves and stay safe, much like an earthquake survivor would respond. One of our basic human needs is to feel safe; to feel safe in the choices we make and feel safe with the healthy control we have in our lives. But the trauma of betrayal takes this away and leaves us feeling unsafe and out of control. In an attempt to stabilize ourselves and our environment, we may develop behaviors that look extreme, when really they are the result of trauma. We become deeply motivated by our need to reestablish safety.

*Partners seek **truth**, not control, though many fail to understand this. A partner's motivation for truth stems from the need to once again feel safe—to keep the environment safe to prevent further trauma and pain.*[21]

In our search for safety and truth, we may unintentionally develop behaviors that are more harmful than helpful, which may interfere with our healing. In this context, think of safety as a condition of being protected from or unlikely to cause danger, risk, or injury. Think of control as the power to influence or direct your own and/or other's behaviors, or the course of events.

---

[20] Barbara Steffens and Marsha Means, *Your Sexually Addicted Spouse: How Partners Can Cope And Heal* (Far Hills: New Horizon Press, 2009), 31.

[21] Steffens and Means, *Your Sexually Addicted Spouse*, 71.

✝ The following table will help you identify what's motivating your behavior. Determine whether it is your need for safety or your need for control, or perhaps both. Check those that apply to you.[22]

BEHAVIOR	Am I seeking Safety?	Am I seeking Control?
01. Checking (Internet, wallet, cell phone)	☐	☐
02. Calling my husband frequently	☐	☐
03. Angry outbursts	☐	☐
04. Obsessing about my husband's behavior	☐	☐
05. Avoiding sexual intimacy	☐	☐
06. Keeping secrets about the addiction	☐	☐
07. Trying to forget about the problem	☐	☐
08. Threatening to leave (or did leave)	☐	☐
09. Participating in my husband's sexual behavior (porn/fantasy)	☐	☐
10. Changing my appearance	☐	☐
11. Giving up things I enjoy so I can be home with my husband	☐	☐
12. Shutting down emotionally/physically	☐	☐
13. Other: _____	☐	☐

[22] Steffens and Means, *Your Sexually Addicted Spouse*, 77

✚ After checking whether your motivation was based on the need for safety and/or control, summarize what you discovered in doing this exercise.

_____

_____

_____

_____

_____

_____

✚ As you look at the chart, can you identify any fears you may be feeling?

_____

_____

_____

_____

_____

_____

When we experience trauma, it affects our brain and body in ways we may not recognize. As with many trauma survivors, they are constantly scanning their environment for threats because their sense of safety has been ripped from them. To someone who doesn't know what they've been through, their behaviors may seem erratic and unpredictable. But to those who understand the effects of trauma, they know what's really going on: a trauma survivor is attempting to recreate a sense of safety in their world. This is also what's happening with a betrayed partner. In the best way they know how, they are recreating what it means to feel safe, despite struggling with the stress and aftershocks of betrayal.

Many women who experienced sexual betrayal identified similar symptoms following discovery/disclosure. This list contains twenty of the most common stress symptoms exhibited following betrayal.[23]

---

[23] Sheri Keffer, *Intimate Deception: Healing the Wounds of Sexual Betrayal* (Grand Rapids: Revell, 2018), 50-51.

✚ **Put a check mark beside each symptom you have or are currently experiencing.**

☐ Shock and disbelief

☐ Anxiety, fear, and/or panic

☐ Emotional arousal and reactivity

☐ Difficulty trusting self and/or others

☐ Withdrawal, detachment, and isolation

☐ Feelings of powerlessness and helplessness

☐ Difficulty concentrating or remembering

☐ Concern about overburdening others with your problems

☐ Emotional numbness and the inability to feel love or joy

☐ Depression, reduced interest in everyday life and activities

☐ Outbursts of irritability, short-temperedness, anger, and rage

☐ Bewilderment, confusion, and the inability to understand what is happening

☐ Alexithymia: the brain goes offline, making it difficult to put words to your feelings

☐ Shame and self-blame, feelings of responsibility for deceptive sexual acts

☐ Preoccupation with body image, undereating, overeating

☐ Worry, intrusive thoughts, reviewing the traumatic details of the discovery

☐ Safety issues, concerns about sexually transmitted diseases or for safety of the children in the home

☐ Fear-induced control, an increased need to control everyday experiences (parenting, childcare, dieting)

☐ Denial, minimizing the experience in order to survive

☐ Hypervigilance, excessive alertness or watchfulness that may look like paranoia but is not and may be mislabeled (by friends, family, pastor, counselor, doctor, etc.)

✚ **Of the symptoms you checked, identify the top three that are creating significant distress and/or disruption in your life. Explain.**

✚ At any point, was there a time when you were responding to the trauma, but not consciously aware of it? Was anyone else involved with bringing it to your attention (safe friend, family member, counselor, or mentor)?

_____

_____

_____

TRAUMA AND THE BRAIN

As with many people who are impacted by trauma, we can be unaware of the extent of our behaviors because our need for safety is foundational to our survival. We may not even recognize that our behaviors are actually a trauma response.

The way betrayal trauma impacts the brain and body can have lasting effects. While each person's situation is different and unique to some extent, research suggests that prolonged exposure to stress and continued perceived threat can create dysregulation of several systems, disrupt functions, and lead to serious forms of psychological trauma.[24] Various regions of the brain, neurotransmitters, hormones, and more are severely impacted by what a betrayed partner is experiencing.

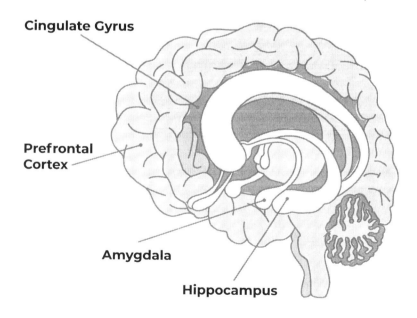

Cingulate Gyrus

Prefrontal Cortex

Amygdala

Hippocampus

[24] Sherin, Jonathan E, and Charles B Nemeroff. "Post-traumatic stress disorder: the neurobiological impact of psychological trauma." _Dialogues in clinical neuroscience_ vol. 13,3 (2011): 263-78. doi:10.31887/DCNS.2011.13.2/jsherin

The **limbic system** is located in the center of the brain—often referred to as the emotional center of the brain. It is not one isolated part of the brain, but rather a collection of structures associated with processing emotion, mood, and memory.[25] The limbic system is made up of several distinct areas, interconnected by their function. Four specific areas of the brain are impacted by trauma.

The **prefrontal cortex**, which interacts with the limbic system, does many amazing things for us: regulates positive and negative emotion, helps with problem-solving, and self-awareness, to name a few.[26] It allows us to apply rational thinking and reasoning to situations, equipping us to make wise decisions.

The **hippocampus** gathers information from many sources—from our environment and life events—and links them together to form memories.[27] It is responsible for consolidating (moving) our short-term memory into long-term memory while we sleep (another reason why sleep is so important).

The **amygdala** regulates our emotional response and assigns meaning based on our environment.[28] Both positive and negative emotions are produced in the amygdala as a result of a rapid assessment of the situation. For example, when someone we love walks into the room, our face will display an emotional response of happiness or pleasure. Or, if someone unexpectedly appears in a dark setting, we may respond with fear because the amygdala has determined that there is a threat or the situation may be dangerous.

When we have an experience, especially an event that is perceived as threatening or dangerous, the hippocampus and the amygdala work together to process the event—the specific details of what happened and the way it made us feel are stored together in our limbic system.

The **cingulate gyrus** helps us to adapt to what's happening around us. It allows us to be flexible and recognize when change is needed.

All of these areas of the brain can be significantly impacted by trauma.

Trauma can have a cascading effect on the normal functioning of our brain and body, causing hyperactivation of some areas of the brain (always in the "on" position), while other areas of the brain become hypoactive (decreased activity). In many ways,

---

25 Peter Abrahams, *How the Brain Works: Understanding Brain Function, Thought, and Personality.* (New York: Metro Books, 2015), 28-29.

26 Tonya Hines, *Anatomy of the Brain*, Mayfield Clinic, 2016, https://mayfieldclinic.com/pe-anatbrain.htm.

27 Daniel J. Siegel, *Pocket Guide to Interpersonal Neurobiology: An Integrative Handbook of the Mind.* (New York: W.W. Norton & Company, Inc., 2012).

28 Peter Abrahams, *How the Brain Works: Understanding Brain Function, Thought, and Personality* (New York: Metro Books, 2015), 28-29.

leaving the brain in a very vulnerable condition.[29] For example, many people who experience trauma tend to have a hyperactive amygdala; it's on high alert, constantly searching for danger. Whereas, their hippocampus becomes hypoactive, disrupting their ability to remember things. It is also during these times of perceived threat that the prefrontal cortex is inhibited, making it more difficult for us to apply rational thought and reason to the situation. And all of these brain areas are influenced by the increase and decrease of chemicals and hormones, creating chaos in the mind and brain of a betrayed partner.

Trauma is perhaps the most avoided, ignored, belittled, denied, misunderstood, and untreated cause of human suffering. Although it is the source of tremendous distress and dysfunction, it is not an ailment or a disease, but the byproduct of an instinctively instigated, altered state of consciousness. We enter this altered state – let us call it "survival mode" – when we perceive that our lives are being threatened. If we are overwhelmed by the threat and are unable to successfully defend ourselves, we can become stuck in survival mode. This highly aroused state is designed solely to enable short-term defensive actions; but left untreated over time, it begins to form the symptoms of trauma.[30]

Our limbic system is always on, searching our environment for danger or perceived threat, so we can quickly respond and survive whatever it is that's threatening to harm us. When we sense danger, our brain and body initiates our Sympathetic Nervous System (SNS) or otherwise referred to as our fight or flight response.[31] This system automatically shuts down various body functions and redirects others, so we have the physical strength and energy to escape danger.

When the danger has passed, our brain and body initiates our Parasympathetic Nervous System (PNS) or otherwise referred to as the rest and digest response. This system helps to bring all our body functions back to normal. It causes us to feel relaxed and calm again because the threat is gone.

Our Sympathetic Nervous System was designed as an alert system. When we sense danger, our body responds, we escape the danger, then we can relax again. This system was never intended to stay in the "ON" position. When this happens, when we are in a situation where we continuously sense danger or feel threatened, it can create a host of physical, mental, and emotional issues.

---

[29] Bremner, J Douglas. "Traumatic stress: effects on the brain." *Dialogues in clinical neuroscience* vol. 8,4 (2006): 445-61. doi:10.31887/DCNS.2006.8.4/jbremner.

[30] Peter Levine, *Waking the Tiger—Healing Trauma: The Innate Capacity to Transform Overwhelming Experiences* (Berkeley: North Atlantic Books, 1997), 23.

[31] Alshak MN, M Das J. Neuroanatomy, Sympathetic Nervous System. [Updated 2021 Jul 26]. In: StatPearls [Internet]. Treasure Island (FL): StatPearls Publishing; 2022 Jan-. Available from: https://www.ncbi.nlm.nih.gov/books/NBK542195/.

And when our limbic system is on high alert and doing its best to help us survive, our prefrontal cortex is inhibited so we lack the ability to apply rational thought and make healthy decisions about our situation. In fact, when we are living in a constant state of stress and trauma from betrayal, it affects our entire body.

The fight-or-flight response itself is meant to be short term and adaptive, which makes sense: When your body goes into that mode, your normal immune function is temporarily shut down. If you think of fight-or-flight as triggered by something like a tiger chasing you, your body devotes energy and resources to running away, not to digesting the last thing you ate — or to sending immune-fighting cells to kill a cold virus. It's when you're in that state chronically that the cascading inflammatory response is set up.

It's this maladaptive response to stress that over time perpetuates itself and becomes implicated in chronic health problems.[32]

+ How has learning about trauma's effect on your brain and behavior been eye opening for you? In what ways has it helped to explain what you've experienced because of betrayal?

+ Since discovery/disclosure, have you experienced any new or increased health concerns?

[32] Denise Schipani, "Here's How Stress and Inflammation Are Linked," *Everyday Health*, October 16, 2018, https://www.everydayhealth.com/wellness/united-states-of-stress/link-between-stress-inflammation/.

While it can be so enlightening to learn how our brain is affected by trauma, it can be even more empowering to understand what this looks like in our behaviors. Based on research, these are common cognitive, emotional, and behavioral responses following betrayal:[33]

Cognitive Responses

- ☐ A sense of victimization
- ☐ Confusion
- ☐ Intense emotions
- ☐ Defensiveness

Emotional Responses

- ☐ Shock
- ☐ Repression
- ☐ Denial
- ☐ Intense mood fluctuations
- ☐ Depression
- ☐ Anxiety
- ☐ Lowered self-esteem

Behavioral Responses

- ☐ Need to repeatedly question the offender
- ☐ Intrusive thoughts about the event
- ☐ Experience hypervigilance
- ☐ Obsessive thoughts

✚ **Check any of the above responses you've experienced following discovery or disclosure. What responses are you currently experiencing or struggling with most?**

_____

_____

_____

_____

_____

_____

_____

Knowing how trauma impacts the brain and body explains what's going on inside us and helps us make sense of our behaviors.[34]

---

[33] Barbara Steffens and Robyn Rennie, "The Traumatic Nature of Disclosure for Wives of Sexual Addicts," _Sexual Addiction & Compulsivity 13_, (2006): 261-263.

[34] If you want more information about how an addict's brain function contributes to their compulsive sexual behaviors, you can jump ahead to the lessons found in Chapter 5 or watch sessions 3, 4, and 7 of the _Sexual Integrity 101_ video course available at **puredesire.org/si101**

God's Grace Trumps Trauma

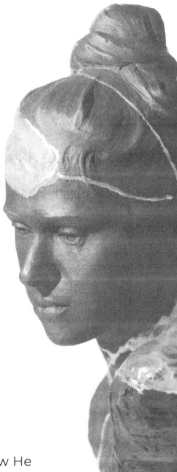

Prior to Jesus' arrest, he was with His disciples, attempting to explain how He would be going away and encouraging them to keep the faith. At one point He says to the disciples:

> *"I have told you all this so that you may have peace in me. Here on earth you will have many trials and sorrows. But take heart, because I have overcome the world."*
>
> JOHN 16:33 (NLT)

This is part of the human experience. We live in a fallen world and, because of this, we will experience various forms of pain and trauma throughout our lives.

No one escapes this; not anyone since the beginning of time. Throughout biblical history, many people have experienced pain and trauma: Adam and Eve; Abraham, Isaac, and Jacob (their wives and children, too); Moses; the Israelites; Joshua; Ruth; David; and the list goes on and on.

The entire Bible—Old and New Testaments—are filled with individual stories of pain, brokenness, and trauma. It's not all little t trauma, but many stories that include significant big T trauma. Anything from lies and deception to affairs, betrayal, and even murder.

This truth is troubling because we can't escape the pain of this life. The good news is that this pain is never wasted in the hands of God. In Exodus 5, when Pharaoh took away the straw for making bricks, the Israelites cried out to God. They thought the solution to their problem was more straw to make bricks. But God had a different plan. He allowed them to experience this hardship because He wanted them to discover that their victory wasn't going to be found in having more straw.

When life is challenging, we can find ourselves crying out to God for more straw: "Lord, I just want some more straw...or more money, or a better job, or a husband who will never struggle with sexual brokenness again! Lord, make this pain go away." When we respond to the pain and troubles of life in this way, it's often an indication that our vision is too focused on the present. To some extent, like the Isrealites, our focus is too narrow and short-sighted. But God can expand our vision to something bigger and take us to an entirely new place—**a place where we find victory in our own journey regardless of our husband's choices.**

The straw was a matter of life or death in the Israelites' minds. From their perspective, it was critical because of the recent trauma Pharaoh had brought into their lives. They were just trying to survive; but God was challenging them to face their fears and pain, and trust Him.

So then the challenge for us: to believe that God has something far better for us than our current situation.

✚ How can you relate to the Israelites and their need for more straw?

_____

_____

_____

✚ Regarding your current situation and the effects of betrayal, in what way has your vision been too small?

_____

_____

_____

✛ If you had a giant vision of what God could do in your current situation and healing, what would that look like? What would you ask God to do in your life?

_____

_____

_____

_____

_____

_____

_____

_____

_____

_____

_____

_____

_____

_____

_____

_____

_____

For many women who have experienced betrayal, their trauma response can be surprising to them and somewhat unexpected. They will likely experience some immediate reactions, as well as some delayed reactions.

The following table highlights several immediate and delayed reactions to trauma within various categories: emotional, physical, cognitive, behavioral, and existential. All of these responses are normal for people who have experienced trauma.

✛ As you read through the immediate and delayed reactions in each category, check the reactions you have experienced or are experiencing since discovery (or disclosure).

Note: If some of your immediate reactions are delayed or some of your delayed reactions are more immediate, it's okay. We all have different life experiences that will contribute to our reactions.

IMMEDIATE AND DELAYED REACTIONS TO TRAUMA[35]

Immediate Emotional Reactions

- ☐ Numbness and detachment
- ☐ Anxiety or severe fear
- ☐ Guilt (including survivor guilt)
- ☐ Exhilaration as a result of surviving
- ☐ Anger
- ☐ Sadness
- ☐ Helplessness
- ☐ Feeling unreal; depersonalization (e.g., feeling as if you are watching yourself)
- ☐ Disorientation
- ☐ Feeling out of control
- ☐ Denial
- ☐ Constriction of feelings
- ☐ Feeling overwhelmed

Delayed Emotional Reactions

- ☐ Irritability and/or hostility
- ☐ Depression
- ☐ Mood swings, instability
- ☐ Anxiety (e.g., phobia, generalized anxiety)
- ☐ Fear of trauma recurrence
- ☐ Grief reactions
- ☐ Shame
- ☐ Feelings of fragility and/or vulnerability
- ☐ Emotional detachment from anything that requires emotional reactions (e.g., significant and/or family relationships, conversations about self, discussion of traumatic events or reactions to them)

Immediate Physical Reactions

- ☐ Nausea and/or gastrointestinal distress
- ☐ Sweating or shivering
- ☐ Faintness
- ☐ Muscle tremors or uncontrollable shaking
- ☐ Elevated heartbeat, respiration, and blood pressure
- ☐ Extreme fatigue or exhaustion
- ☐ Greater startle responses
- ☐ Depersonalization

Delayed Physical Reactions

- ☐ Sleep disturbances, nightmares
- ☐ Somatization (e.g., increased focus on and worry about body aches/pains)
- ☐ Appetite and digestive changes
- ☐ Lowered resistance to colds and infection
- ☐ Persistent fatigue
- ☐ Elevated cortisol levels
- ☐ Hyperarousal
- ☐ Long-term health effects including heart, liver, autoimmune, and chronic obstructive pulmonary disease

---

[35] Center for Substance Abuse Treatment (US). Trauma-Informed Care in Behavioral Health Services. Rockville (MD): Substance Abuse and Mental Health Services Administration (US); 2014. (Treatment Improvement Protocol (TIP) Series, No. 57.) Exhibit 1.3-1, Immediate and Delayed Reactions to Trauma. Available from: https://www.ncbi.nlm.nih.gov/books/NBK207191/table/part1_ch3.t1/.

Immediate Cognitive Reactions

- ☐ Difficulty concentrating
- ☐ Rumination or racing thoughts (e.g., replaying the traumatic event over and over again)
- ☐ Distortion of time and space (e.g., traumatic event may be perceived as if it was happening in slow motion, or a few seconds can be perceived as minutes)
- ☐ Memory problems (e.g., not being able to recall important aspects of the trauma)
- ☐ Strong identification with victims

Delayed Cognitive Reactions

- ☐ Intrusive memories or flashbacks
- ☐ Reactivation of previous traumatic events
- ☐ Self-blame
- ☐ Preoccupation with event
- ☐ Difficulty making decisions
- ☐ Magical thinking: belief that certain behaviors, including avoidant behavior, will protect against future trauma
- ☐ Belief that feelings or memories are dangerous
- ☐ Generalization of triggers (e.g., a person who experiences a home invasion during the daytime may avoid being alone during the day)
- ☐ Suicidal thinking

Immediate Behavioral Reactions

- ☐ Startled reaction
- ☐ Restlessness
- ☐ Sleep and appetite disturbances
- ☐ Difficulty expressing oneself
- ☐ Argumentative behavior
- ☐ Increased use of alcohol, drugs, and tobacco
- ☐ Withdrawal and apathy
- ☐ Avoidant behaviors

Delayed Behavioral Reactions

- ☐ Avoidance of event reminders
- ☐ Social relationship disturbances
- ☐ Decreased activity level
- ☐ Engagement in high-risk behaviors
- ☐ Increased use of alcohol and drugs
- ☐ Withdrawal

Immediate Existential Reactions

- ☐ Intense use of prayer
- ☐ Restoration of faith in the goodness of others (e.g., receiving help from others)

Delayed Existential Reactions

- ☐ Questioning (e.g., "Why me?")
- ☐ Increased cynicism, disillusionment
- ☐ Increased self-confidence (e.g., "If I can survive this, I can survive anything")

- [ ] Loss of self-efficacy
- [ ] Immediate disruption of life assumptions (e.g., fairness, safety, goodness, predictability of life)

- [ ] Loss of purpose
- [ ] Renewed faith
- [ ] Hopelessness
- [ ] Reestablishing priorities
- [ ] Redefining meaning and importance of life
- [ ] Reworking life's assumptions to accommodate the trauma (e.g., taking a self-defense class to reestablish a sense of safety)

✚ **Of the immediate reactions you marked, which are most surprising or unexpected to you?**

_____

_____

_____

_____

_____

_____

_____

_____

_____

✚ **List the top five immediate reactions you're struggling with today.**

01. _____

02. _____

03. _____

04. _____

05. _____

+ Of the delayed reactions you marked, which are most surprising or unexpected to you?

_____

_____

_____

_____

+ List the top five delayed reactions you're struggling with today.

01. _____

02. _____

03. _____

04. _____

05. _____

Betrayal trauma creates real physical and emotional responses. It creates chaos in our brain and body. We may be crying one minute and angry the next! We may not have words to express what we're feeling. We might not even **know** what we're feeling! Since we have been lied to, manipulated, and deceived for so long, we may struggle with trusting others. Our need for safety can make us more guarded and protective about our environment, even to the point of being unable to let go of any control because we cannot risk being hurt again.

These responses are not intentionally malicious, but rather a means of trying to feel safe and survive the after-effects of betrayal. We can become so focused on our situation and our need to protect ourselves, that we lose sight of this important fact: our heavenly Father is with us, no matter where we are, no matter what we're going through. He can be trusted and will never leave us.

This is why praising God encourages and strengthens us as we go through difficult situations; worship declares the truth of who God is in the midst of our pain and trauma. More than ever, we need to hear from God and praise Him, trusting Him for revelation and breakthrough. We have to choose to not be controlled by the pain and trauma created through betrayal.

We serve a Lord who understands our pain and heartache. He knows what we're going through. When we take our eyes off our current situation and focus on Him, He will bring healing to our heart, mind, and body.

> *Therefore, as you have received Christ Jesus the Lord, so walk in Him, having been firmly rooted and now being built up in Him and established in your faith, just as you were instructed, and overflowing with gratitude.*
>
> COLOSSIANS 2:6-7 (NASB)

We will not only be able to stand on a firm foundation that comes through our relationship with Him, but He will build us up and comfort us throughout this process.

> *All praise to God, the Father of our Lord Jesus Christ. God is our merciful Father and the source of all comfort. He comforts us in all our troubles so that we can comfort others. When they are troubled, we will be able to give them the same comfort God has given us.*
>
> 2 CORINTHIANS 1:3-4 (NLT)

Our heavenly Father will comfort us exactly where we're at; and after we have received His gracious healing in our lives, He will provide an opportunity for us to comfort others. He will transform our pain and trauma into a beautiful story of hope and redemption. Then, when we share our story of healing with other women who are going through the heartbreak of betrayal, it will encourage and comfort them. Like the women in this group, when we take the brave step to embark on this healing journey, the Holy Spirit will do a miraculous work in our lives.

✛ **What thoughts and feelings do you have about God using your healing to provide hope and encouragement to other women who've experienced betrayal?**

If we want God to sovereignly heal our pain and trauma, we need to embrace these four concepts as we continue on our journey.

1. The trial you are going through will facilitate God's purpose in your life.

The trauma and pain you're experiencing, God did not cause this; but **God promises to redeem it and use it for His purpose and good.** Everything that has happened can be used by the hand of God, if you trust Him with it. Only a sovereign God can take the messiness of our lives and transform it into something beautiful; something that reflects His grace and goodness in our lives.

2. Don't deny your pain, trauma, and points of betrayal.

As you continue going through these lessons, you may have to stop at some point and grieve. It will help you prepare for the future lessons by grieving what was taken from you because of your husband's addiction. It is important to express how you feel about the pain and trauma you are experiencing because of the betrayal. While this may be challenging, it will benefit you to face this heartache and identify what you've lost in this process.

3. Recognize how God's grace trumps all your trauma.

God is devastated that this has happened to us—that any of us would experience betrayal—but He will always find ways to use our pain. He doesn't waste it. He redeems it. God may be using your current situation to raise you up with great authority to reach many women who are hurting from betrayal. He may be uniquely equipping you to help others. You understand how it feels to face the hurt and trauma of sexual betrayal. All of this is evidence of God's grace in this process. God's grace is what transforms you from a wounded woman to an empowered advocate, committed to your own healing and ready to help others in their healing journey.

4. Learn to live "heart-to-heart."

As we walk out our healing and discover what healthy relationships look like, we will become skilled at living "heart-to-heart" with others. We will no longer live in pain or live out of our woundedness, but live through God's healing grace in our lives: loving others exactly where they're at; coming alongside, supporting, and encouraging other women who've experienced betrayal; sharing our story of pain, grief, and injustice, and the hope that comes with healing.

✚ Of these four concepts, which one is most challenging for you right now?

_____
_____
_____
_____
_____
_____
_____
_____
_____
_____

✚ Which of these four concepts is most encouraging to you right now?

_____
_____
_____
_____
_____
_____
_____
_____
_____
_____

Loosening Trauma's Hold

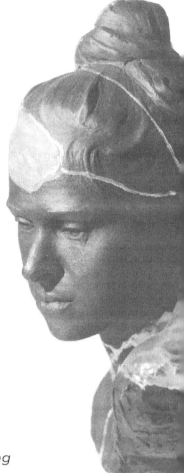

I don't know what to do? Since discovering my fiancee's addiction to pornography, it feels like I'm forced to make decisions with no good outcomes. Either I stay with him, knowing this will be a part of our life together, or I leave the relationship. And even though we're in counseling right now, it's definitely a two steps forward, one step back process.

Like last week, when he relapsed again. Initially, I was flooded with all the same feelings I had with discovery and wanted to run away. We were able to talk through it, which helped me to calm down, but my mind continued to race, weighing the pros and cons of this relationship. I continue to ask myself, "What will it cost me if I stay? What will it cost me if I leave?"

CAMILA

✚ **Can you relate to how Camila is feeling? Explain.**

_____

_____

_____

_____

_____

Dealing with trauma in our lives creates a **Double Bind**; a lose-lose predicament we face.[36] **If we choose to ignore the effects of betrayal, it can pile up and affect us physically, emotionally, and spiritually.** It is literally like trying to pull your fingers out of Chinese handcuffs. The harder you pull away, the worse it gets. So it is when we attempt to ignore our pain and trauma; the impact it has on us only gets worse.

The other option to this Double Bind is to face the fear of dealing with our pain— the pain we have tried to ignore. The only way to get out of the Chinese handcuffs is to push your fingers farther into the tube to the point where the straw strips actually expand out in width and release their hold.[37] **Our intuitive reaction is to pull away—yet God says we have to press into the place of discomfort and pain to be released from it.**

Thankfully, when we choose to face the pain and pursue healing, the Holy Spirit is advocating for us:

> *In the same way, the Spirit helps us in our weakness. We do not know what we ought to pray for, but the Spirit himself intercedes for us through wordless groans. And he who searches our hearts knows the mind of the Spirit, because the Spirit intercedes for God's people in accordance with the will of God.*
>
> ROMANS 8:26-27 (NIV)

The Holy Spirit graciously intercedes for us. It is the gracious nature of God at work, deep within our soul, that will enable us to overcome our fear and press into the pain and trauma created through betrayal.

✝ **How do you feel, knowing that the Holy Spirit is interceding for you through this healing process?**

_____

_____

_____

_____

_____

_____

_____

---

[36] Michael Dye, *The Genesis Process for Change Groups, Book One* (Auburn: Michael Dye, 2006), 45-52.

[37] Victoria M. Follette and Jacqueline Pistorello, *Finding Life Beyond Trauma* (Canada: Raincoast Books, 2007), 98.

When we courageously face the pain of our trauma, it will be challenging at times, but will also help us recognize when we're living in trauma.

Living In Trauma

When we are living with trauma—living with the residual effects of a traumatic experience—it takes a toll on us in ways we may not recognize. While we are motivated by our need for safety and think we're navigating our situation in a healthy way, it may actually be hurting us in the long run.

One study revealed symptoms of trauma among practicing Christians.[38]

- ☐ Sleep disturbances/nightmares about the event
- ☐ Becoming very anxious when something reminds you of the event
- ☐ Replaying or reliving the event over and over in your mind
- ☐ Avoiding thought or memories related to the trauma
- ☐ Grief or a sense of loss
- ☐ Avoiding reminders of the event (avoiding places, people, activities, etc.)
- ☐ Having strong negative feelings such as anger, fear, horror
- ☐ Always on alert or on guard; feeling jumpy
- ☐ Loss of interest in activities you used to enjoy
- ☐ Shame or guilt
- ☐ Feeling like no one is listening to you / you've lost your voice
- ☐ Withdrawing from family or friends
- ☐ A feeling of helplessness that lasted more than just a few weeks
- ☐ Trouble experiencing feelings (unable to feel happiness / love)
- ☐ Unable to eat or overeating
- ☐ Irritable behavior, angry outbursts, or aggressive behavior
- ☐ Experiencing physical symptoms when thinking about the event
- ☐ Negative behaviors (alcohol / substance abuse, self-harm, etc.)

✚ Since discovery (or disclosure) of your husband's sexual addiction, have you experienced any of these trauma symptoms? Put a check mark next to those you've experienced and are true for you.

---

[38] American Bible Society, *Trauma In America: Understanding How People Face Hardships and How the Church Offers Hope* (Ventura: Barna Group, 2020), 23.

✚ **What thoughts and feelings do you have about the symptoms you marked as true for you? Explain.**

_____

_____

_____

_____

_____

Psychologists usually try to help people use insight and understanding to manage their behavior. However, neuroscience research shows that very few psychological problems are the result of defects in understanding; most originate in pressures from deeper regions in the brain that drive our perception and attention. When the alarm bell of the emotional brain keeps signaling that you are in danger, no amount of insight will silence it.[39]

✚ **How does this quote relate to what you've experienced through betrayal?**

_____

_____

_____

_____

This quote is so true for those who experience betrayal. It seems as though an alarm is going off in our brain, warning us of danger. We become hypervigilant: constantly scanning our environment for threat. We can't sleep. We can't eat. Our mind replays these traumatic events over and over, trying to make sense of what's happening. It is relentless.

In the previously mentioned study revealing symptoms of trauma among practicing Christians, they found that 52% struggled with sleep disturbances, 49% struggled with anxiety, and 49% struggled with ruminating about the traumatic event.[40] This

---

[39] Bessel van der Kolk, *The Body Keeps the Score: Brain, Mind, and Body in the Healing of Trauma* (New York: Penguin Books, 2014), 64.

[40] American Bible Society, *Trauma In America, Understanding How People Face Hardships and How the Church Offers Hope* (Ventura: Barna Group, 2020), 22.

reinforces the fact that trauma can have lasting effects on our brain, body, and soul. It also points to why we work so hard to reestablish a sense of safety in our lives after experiencing betrayal. When our lives have been turned upside down, having a sense of authority over your own life is important.

✚ Describe a situation that felt unsafe, in which you feared the outcome if you did not take control. Explain.

✚ What was the outcome of this situation?

✚ What things give you a sense of healthy control in your life?

Healing and Attachment

As we learn to recognize how trauma is affecting us, it can be helpful to understand how our attachment style or an attachment injury may be interfering with our healing.

Attachment refers to our ability to bond with others.[41] As infants, we depend on others to meet our needs and keep us safe. When our needs are consistently met in a safe environment, we tend to develop a secure attachment style. However, when our needs are neglected, and our environment feels scary and confusing, we are more likely to develop an insecure attachment style.

Our attachment style plays a significant role in how we relate to others in our adult relationships; not only intimate relationships, but all relationships. Our attachment style reflects how we learned to be in relationships and forms the foundation for how we behave in relationships.

Based on research, several leading psychologists have determined that there are four types of attachment styles.[42] While this description is not exhaustive, it provides common characteristics found within each type.[43]

Secure:

- Easily develops relationships with others.
- Comfortable depending on others and being depended upon for support.
- Healthy balance between independence and connectedness.
- Relaxed, present, and playful in relationships.
- Practices repair; easily recovers from conflict.

Avoidant:

- Disconnected and closed-off in relationships.
- Lacks a sense of belonging.
- Finds intimate relationships distressing.
- Unable to emotionally connect.
- Prefers isolation.

---

[41] Diane Poole Heller, Understanding Attachment Styles and Their Effect on Relationships, February 7, 2022, https://dianepooleheller.com/understanding-attachment-styles-and-their-effect-on-relationships/.

[42] Kendra Cherry, What Is Attachment Theory? The Importance of Early Emotional Bonds, Verywell Mind, July 17, 2019, https://www.verywellmind.com/what-is-attachment-theory-2795337.

[43] Diane Poole Heller, *Adult Attachment Styles Reference Guide*, Trauma Solutions, 2022.

Ambivalent

- Craves connection, yet pushes others away.
- Fears abandonment and finds it difficult to trust others.
- Lacks self-care and the ability to self-soothe.
- Negatively misinterprets cues.
- Separation is distressing.

Disorganized

- Wants close relationships, but fears it at the same time.
- Difficulty trusting others; views relationships as dangerous.
- Extreme dysregulation, often appearing chaotic.
- Acts out in confusing ways.
- Sudden mood shifts.

Our attachment style is developed early in life because it's directly tied to our survival and our ability to feel safe in our environment. Even if we have a secure attachment style, when something happens in our relationship, creating a sense that we are not safe or in danger, it threatens our attachment and interferes with the connection we have with the other person in the relationship. This is what betrayal does in our relationship. In fact, research suggests that when infidelity happens, creating an attachment injury, the betrayed partner will likely exhibit disorganized attachment behaviors.[44] This is because an insecure attachment style—Avoidant, Ambivalent, and Disorganized—shares similar behavioral characteristics to those exhibited by people who have experienced trauma. The trauma experienced through betrayal may manifest itself as an insecure attachment style.

✚ **Based on the above characteristics, what type of attachment style do you have? Keep in mind, you may see yourself within several types, which is common.**

---

[44] Benjamin Warach and Lawrence Josephs, "The aftershocks of infidelity: a review of infidelity-based attachment trauma," *Sexual and Relationship Therapy*, 36 (2019): 68-90.

✚ How has your attachment style changed because of betrayal ? Explain.

_____

_____

_____

_____

_____

_____

_____

_____

_____

Exploring our attachment style helps us to make sense of our relationship trauma. Even if we have sustained an attachment injury because of betrayal, the work we do to find healing will help us to get back to a secure form of attachment.

Being comfortable in your own skin and having tools that help you relax is a really big deal, but learning how to feel safe with others is revolutionary. When your nervous system can co-regulate with other people, and you feel safe and playful and relaxed, you can develop a stronger sense of secure attachment and enjoy its profound rewards...[45]

Co-regulation refers to the way we interact with others and our ability to adjust ourselves in order to appropriately maintain our emotions.[46] When we are in close relationship with others, our emotional awareness and stability allows us to influence the emotional state of the other person. In the same way, we are also influenced by another's emotional response, which can be helpful during times of stress. Co-regulation describes the interaction between two people, the back and forth exchange between them, both adjusting their emotional response based on the response of the other.

This is great news! Healing our trauma provides the opportunity to grow and change in all areas of our lives, even our attachment style. And we do this best when we are in a safe and supportive community. Especially while our primary relationship isn't secure, it's important to be in a community with healthy people.

---

[45] Diane Poole Heller, _The Power of Attachment: How to Create Deep and Lasting Intimate Relationships_ (Boulder: Sounds True, 2019), 7-8.

[46] David Belford, _Co-Regulation and Self-Regulation_, Center for Development and Disability, The University of New Mexico, February 2012.

✚ **How are you encouraged through learning about your attachment style and how it contributes to your healing?**

_____

_____

_____

_____

_____

_____

_____

_____

_____

_____

_____

_____

_____

_____

_____

_____

_____

_____

_____

As we process our pain and trauma, it will no longer hold us hostage, creating chaos in our brain and body. Healing from betrayal frees us to become the person God created us to be.

Note: If you are feeling triggered by any of the lesson content or this healing process, and want to pursue professional help, please contact Pure Desire at 503-489-0230 or visit **puredesire.org/counseling**.

3

CHAPTER THREE

What Does My Healing Journey Look Like ?

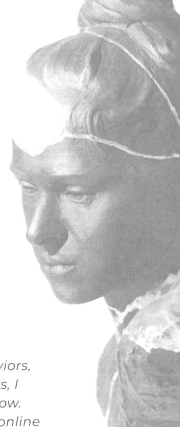

The Stages of Healing

When my husband finally disclosed about his compulsive sexual behaviors, there was a part of me that immediately felt vindicated. For a few years, I knew something was off but I couldn't figure out what it was. Now I know. Not only had he been using pornography, but had begun to dabble in online chats and other acting out behaviors.

At first, my emotions bounced around like a pinball, one minute feeling angry and vengeful, then feeling extremely depressed and hopeless. I would keep myself super busy, in an attempt to outrun and avoid my feelings about all of this. But the minute I slowed down, my thoughts and feelings would overwhelm me. For several months, I cried myself to sleep each night.

I've joined a support group with other women who have experienced betrayal. It has been amazing to have my feelings validated and it continues to help me see the value of my own healing. When I let myself feel the extent of my pain, it feels like I've lost a loved one. But I haven't. It's strange to grieve a life you thought you had.

My husband wants to make plans for our future, and I'm still trying to figure out if we have a future together. I don't know if I will ever trust him again. Right now, I'm focusing on my healing. Taking it one day at a time.

ISABELLA

_____

_____

_____

_____

_____

_____

The Healing Process for a Betrayed Partner

While the stages of healing from betrayal are common to some extent, the way each partner processes through the stages will be specific to their situation. These stages were originally developed by Dr. Patrick Carnes, based on research done with partners of sex addicts, which describe their progression over a five year period.[1]

- Stage 1: Developing/Pre-Discovery
- Stage 2: Crisis/Decision/Information Gathering
- Stage 3: Shock
- Stage 4: Grief/Ambivalence
- Stage 5: Repair
- Stage 6: Growth

For some, you may be able to clearly see what stage you are at today. For others, you may be within a couple stages. Some partners spend months in one stage or cycle through the stages quickly. There may be times when something happens that triggers you back to a previous stage (especially if there is a relapse or new discovery/disclosure), where you may not stay long, but it will take you through a deeper healing experience. Your situation is unique to you and so will be the process by which you experience these stages.

For many partners, understanding these stages gives them hope; knowing they are

---

[1] Stefanie Carnes, _Mending a Shattered Heart: A Guide for Partners of Sex Addicts_ (Carefree: Gentle Path Press, 2011), 42-52.

not alone and that the pain they feel today will not last forever.

Here is a brief snapshot of each stage.

STAGE 1: DEVELOPING/PRE-DISCOVERY

During this stage, you are likely unaware of what's going on. Without knowing it, you may have witnessed your husband attempting to manage his addictive behaviors: working late, unexplained lapses in time, lack of family engagement, unexplained financial loss, and more. Even if you had some indication of your husband's pornography use (or other compulsive sexual behaviors), you probably don't know the extent of his hidden behaviors. This stage may last months or years, where you question some of his behaviors and sense that something's not right, but you believe his lies.

STAGE 2: CRISIS/DECISION/ INFORMATION GATHERING

This stage is initiated by the discovery or disclosure of your husband's secret life. The crisis this creates is life-changing. If you respond to crisis by withdrawing, you may strive to keep the peace, not wanting to know anything more about your husband's behaviors, wanting to focus on your normal responsibilities. If you respond to crisis more proactively, you may require honesty and accountability from your husband, becoming a detective to determine if he is still acting out. Trust is broken and you are hurting. You want information so you can get help for your husband.

STAGE 3: SHOCK

There is often overlap between stages 2 and 3. In the midst of the initial crisis, making decisions, and learning more about sex addiction, you are in shock. The feeling of betrayal is overwhelming, trust no longer exists in the relationship, and you don't know what to believe. You experience times of numbness and tears, followed by anger, shame, and hostility. This may last for months. Having the outside voice of a counselor and/or support group will help to validate your pain, minimize your self-doubt, and break through the isolation that surrounds addiction and the trauma of betrayal.

STAGE 4: GRIEF/AMBIVALENCE

One of the most important steps in the healing process is moving through your pain and experiencing grief. Many betrayed partners will feel a host of emotions: anger, pain, sadness, rejection, and more. Anger is considered a secondary emotion, often covering pain and sadness. As you process through your anger and address the grief you're experiencing, identifying your losses is an important step in this stage. You may begin to feel ambivalent about the relationship. It is often during this stage that you grow in self-awareness, focusing on your needs, and making your healing a priority.

STAGE 5: REPAIR

This stage is characterized by an increased self-awareness and less focus on your husband's behavior. This is also when you may recognize some connections between the betrayal you've experienced and other types of trauma in your life. Many partners will experience a deeper level of spirituality. Your involvement in a support group will strengthen your coping skills, help you set healthy boundaries, and provide emotional stability.

STAGE 6: GROWTH

This stage reflects continued transformation. Many partners let go of feeling victimized and embrace resiliency. Their suffering has been replaced with meaning and purpose. While this process was challenging, you recognize that your husband's addiction was the catalyst for this life-changing experience. You want to help others find hope after betrayal. You have replaced old patterns with new, healthy patterns. You face life head-on with clarity, confidence, and a greater commitment to your healing.

✚ Based on these brief descriptions, where are you in these stages? Explain.

✚ **What encouragement and hope for the future does Stage 6 give you?**

_____

_____

_____

_____

_____

_____

_____

_____

_____

_____

_____

One of the most challenging aspects of the recovery and healing process is that rarely are both spouses at the same place at the same time. Especially, when they are first getting started, it can feel like they are miles apart.

It is common for the addict to get into counseling and/or a recovery group first, since they are clearly the one with the most distressing issues. However, some partners think that once their husband figures out his issues, life will go back to normal. What they don't initially realize is that as their husband begins to experience some honesty, accountability, and relationship with others, they feel relief. Their secret is out! They are getting help. They no longer have to hang their head in shame when walking into church. They are on the path to recovery!

And what does this do for the betrayed partner? Oftentimes, she feels hurt, angry, and is in disbelief. She thinks: _He shouldn't be so happy. He's the one who did this. Doesn't he know how much pain I'm in?_

This is why it's so important for both spouses to be in recovery and support groups (if you choose to stay in the relationship and if your husband is willing to work on his recovery). At Pure Desire, you will often hear the phrase, "Trust the process." It's so true! If you are early in this process, there may be times when the pace will feel agonizingly slow. Because we don't know what we don't know. But if we trust the process, knowing that so many men and women have successfully gone through it, it helps us to stay the course. And at some point, many couples end up at the same place, pursuing health and wholeness together.

✚ When considering the healing process, do you think you are at the same place or at a different place than your husband? Explain.

_____

_____

_____

_____

_____

_____

_____

_____

_____

_____

_____

_____

_____

_____

Many professionals who work in recovery and healing often describe this journey as a 3-5 year process. While this may seem daunting, it doesn't mean your spouse will still be in the throes of his addiction this entire time. It often takes 3-5 years for both the betrayed partner and her spouse to rewire their brains and create a healthy relationship. Some professionals have seen this play out in their work with couples. Carol Juergensen Sheets, a counselor who works with couples, has observed this timeline when it comes to repairing the relationship:[2]

- The first 9-12 months for the couple to learn the tools;

- the next 18-24 months for the couple to sync and use the tools regularly in their daily lives;

- the next 3-5 years for the couple to recalibrate, when they are both doing the work and pursuing their own healing.

---

[2] Carol Juergensen Sheets, _Disclosure Trauma_, Multidimensional Partner Trauma Model Training, Day 2, June 12, 2021, The Association of Partners of Sex Addicts Trauma Specialists (APSATS).

✚ **What are your thoughts and feelings about this timeline?**

_____

_____

_____

_____

_____

_____

_____

_____

✚ **What is encouraging about this timeline?**

_____

_____

_____

_____

_____

_____

_____

_____

_____

Healing from betrayal trauma is possible. It requires consistent, intentional work which may be challenging at times, yet will yield a beautiful transformation of your heart, mind, and soul.

As Scripture tells us, when we live covered in God's grace, it helps us to become more Christlike. Not living a perfect life, but focused on His will and doing what pleases Him.

For the grace of God has appeared that offers salvation to all people. It teaches us to say "No" to ungodliness and worldly passions, and to live self-controlled, upright and godly lives in this present age,

TITUS 2:11-12 (NIV)

✝ In what areas is it easy to apply God's grace in your life?

✝ In what areas is it difficult to apply God's grace in your life?

Grace is one of the main anchors we all need to apply to our lives. Being involved in this support group will help you anchor yourself and your healing in God's grace.

Lifting the Mask to Heal the Wounds

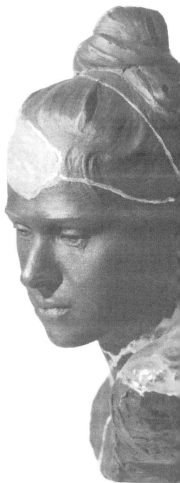

I never intended to hide the real me from the world. It seemed to happen over time, even before I knew the extent of my husband's sexual addiction. We would fight about where he had been or why he had to "work late" some nights, sometimes arguing even as we pulled into the church parking lot. But then the car doors would open and we put on a happy face. We "appeared" to be a loving couple, who had the perfect marriage, and served in church regularly. But this was not the truth.

For me, putting on a happy face or serving in church was a way of masking how I really felt. It was a way of protecting how I really felt about myself and my situation. If I could convince others I was doing great, maybe it would help to convince myself. I wanted to be real, but didn't want others to see how much I was hurting.

MIA

✚ **What parts of Mia's story resonate with you?**

_____

_____

_____

_____

_____

_____

_____

_____

_____

_____

_____

_____

Creating masks is part of our fallen nature. It started in the Garden of Eden when God asked Adam, "Where are you?" Have you noticed that God asks questions hoping we will figure out what is going on. Adam's response is:

> _"I heard you in the garden and I was afraid because I was naked. And I hid."_
> GENESIS 3:10 (MSG)

Adam and Eve fashioned the first masks out of leaves in an attempt to hide their shame, embarrassment, and fear over what they had done. Masks can also be fashioned to cover what has been done to us (i.e. betrayal, abuse, abandonment, or rejection).

Masks hide our insecurities and give us a false feeling that we are in control. We wear masks not because we are evil, but because we are wounded. The enemy exploits our pain and we believe the lies he has deposited in our brain. By wearing masks, our hope is that this sophisticated facade will bring us acceptance and love we all desperately need. When we believe the lies the enemy has spoken to us, our immediate response is to hide.

In evaluating my own behaviors, I realized I had worn masks because of my distorted beliefs about myself: mine included the Pleaser, Performance, Perfectionist, and Take Charge masks. We all wear masks to protect ourselves. We fear the rejection that could happen if people really knew us or knew what happened to us.

✚ **What do you hide behind your masks? Check the masks with which you can identify.**[3]

MASK	DISTORTED BELIEFS
☐ Self-sufficient mask	People may need me but I don't need anyone.
☐ Fortress mask	Protects me from getting close to people who could hurt me.
☐ Take Charge mask	I have to be in control so I won't get hurt.
☐ Superior mask	If I look better than others, I will be accepted.
☐ Victim mask	Everyone is trying to hurt me.
☐ Party mask	I have to be the life of the party to be accepted.
☐ Pleaser mask	I can't say "no" because I will be liked only if I am needed.
☐ Vanity mask	My value comes from my outward appearance.
☐ Rescuer mask	I am responsible for others' problems, feelings, or behaviors.
☐ Performance mask	My value is based on my performance and how well I measure up.
☐ Happy mask	People only like me when I am happy and fun to be with.
☐ "I Can Do It" mask	Asking for help is a sign of weakness.
☐ Perfectionist mask	I won't be liked if I make mistakes.
☐ Other: _____	
☐ Other: _____	

---

[3] Rebecca Bradley and Diane Roberts, *Behind the Mask* (Gresham: Pure Desire Ministries International, 2012), 14.

✚ List the top five masks you have used to protect yourself. Next to each you listed, share what its job was and how it protected you.

THE MASK   Its job – How did it protect you ?

_____

_____

_____

_____

_____

✚ What have you experienced as a result of wearing these masks ?

_____

_____

_____

_____

_____

✚ How have these masks helped or hindered your life ?

_____

_____

_____

_____

_____

Not only do masks take a lot of energy to maintain, but they literally suffocate the beauty of who God created us to be. Wearing masks also creates an inability to discover our uniqueness because we are trying to be someone we're not. The very parts of us we are trying to hide—our weaknesses, hurts, pains, and trauma—are the very places God wants to do His next miracle. In his New Testament letters to the early Christian church, the Apostle Paul often talked about his weaknesses. He declares that at those very places of weakness, God wanted to bring strength to his life.

The very thing we are desperately seeking—unconditional love, acceptance, and a sense of belonging—actually become unattainable when we put on a mask. The feelings of emptiness continue because only the mask receives what we're seeking. People will compliment our "performance" (mask) or whatever we have done to "please" (mask), but not the person who we really are underneath the mask. Deep down we fear, *If they knew what happened to me, they wouldn't love or accept me.* And when people compliment the mask, rather than us, it personally reinforces the lie we believe about ourselves.

When it comes to healing from betrayal trauma, it may not be safe for a partner to be transparent—remove her masks—in some situations and relationships; those that may require a level of continued self-protection. One of the goals of this healing journey is to find relationships, with God and others, where we can safely remove our masks.

Keep your eyes open this week as you observe the use of masks: not only the masks you wear but the masks other people in your life wear to cover up their insecurities. Try to identify times when your feelings on the inside do not match up with what you are expressing on the outside. When you can identify the masks you wear, you can intentionally allow the Lord to speak His unconditional grace into the hurting parts of your heart.[4]

✚ In the space below, identify the masks you wore during the week, as well as any you noticed that were worn by others. Explain one situation where you wore a mask this week and why you felt it was necessary.

[4] Bradley and Roberts, *Behind the Mask*, 15-16.

The next lesson will help us understand how we can heal those parts of us we have so diligently tried to hide behind the masks we wear.

REVEALING YOUR TRUE SELF

If you have ever been to a circus or a fair, chances are you have seen some of the funny warped mirrors. I remember when our children were quite young how they loved walking in front of the mirror that made them look short and wide, but their favorite was the one that stretched their bodies to look taller than Mom! We'd laugh because we knew they weren't real.

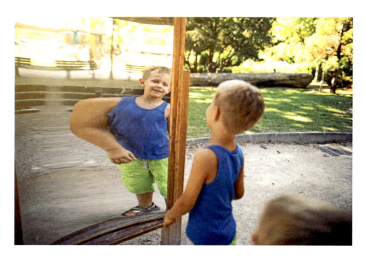

Sadly, the enemy uses warped mirrors in our lives to convince us, "There is something wrong with me, I am defective" or "If people knew what had happened to me, they would reject me." The origin of these lies often comes from the trauma we've experienced. When we feel shame from painful events in our lives, our immediate emotional response is to create a mask.

However, when we become more self-aware, we recognize we have a choice to make: am I going to continue to believe the warped mirror the enemy has been holding up or am I going to believe who God created me to be?

CHANGING MIRRORS:

✚ Step one is identify the lies the enemy has used to try to destroy who God created you to be. In the mirror that follows, write down the lies the enemy has created in your brain due to betrayal.

You can look back at your trauma of infringement/abandonment table (Chapter 2, Lesson 1) and think about the lies that might be attached to those traumatic experiences.

Mirror held up by Satan

Example: I have to be perfect to get love

01. _____

02. _____

03. _____

04. _____

05. _____

✚ Step two is to replace Satan's lies with GOD'S truths about you. How do you do this ?

From the very beginning in the garden with Adam and Eve, the enemy has tried to put a mantle of shame on all of us. But Jesus changed everything when He went to another garden: The Garden of Gethsemane (which means "oil press"). If you go to this garden today, you will see olive trees that Christ might have knelt next to while praying, as some of the trees are over 2,000 years old. In this garden, Christ made the decision to reverse the curse and chose to be crucified, so that He could hold up a new mirror and proclaim who He created you to be. We are made in His image (Gen. 1:26-27) and by going to the cross, He was reclaiming who you really are and who God created you to be. Jesus paid the price for the new mirror. Hebrews 12:2 (NKJV) proclaims:

> *...who for the joy that was set before Him endured the cross, despising the shame, and has sat down at the right hand of the throne of God.*

Christ not only died for our sin, but also despised (one translation says "refused") every bit of shame the enemy has tried to attach to us. I love Charlie Shedd's prayer: **"Lord, help me to understand what you had in mind when you made the original me."**[5]

✚ Write Charlie Shedd's prayer replacing "me" with your name.

Lord help...

_____

_____

_____

_____

[5] Joanna Weaver, *Having a Mary Spirit: Allowing God to Change Us From the Inside Out* (Colorado Springs: Waterbrook Press, 2008), 234.

In the past, maybe you tried to memorize Scripture, proclaiming the truth of who you are in Christ, and yet the lies continually come back to haunt you. Why didn't it work? Part of the reason is that you did a left brain exercise, expecting a right brain response. You applied logical information to the lies. But, the lies originate in the emotional part of your brain.

When we take time to sit quietly before the Lord and allow His Spirit to speak to us, He will reveal great things to us. And it's often through this type of process that we experience God; where He speaks a personal word to us, about us, declaring how He sees us. When this happens, it is a very personal and emotional encounter with God (a right brain experience) and can result in God giving us a personal word (a *rhema* word, a revelation word). Then after receiving this personal word from God, we can find a Scripture, or a *logos* word (a left brain truth) that validates God's revealed truth to us.

I love what Neil Anderson says: **"No person can consistently behave in a way that is inconsistent with the way he perceives himself."**[6] If I believe "I will never be enough" or "I'll never measure up" my behavior will end up being consistent with my self-perception. In order to replace the lie with the truth, you need to have a new experience to impact your limbic system.

> **Limbic Lies are only changed through new and opposite experiences.**

For healing to take place the brain needs to be reprogrammed through new and opposite experiences.

> 66 *Effective healing...must be experiential. It takes an opposite healing experience from the hurt to change the heart.*[7]

In light of Charlie Shedd's prayer that you wrote for yourself, use the mirror that follows to begin declaring **who God created you to be**.

Take each lie you wrote in the warped mirror and replace it with who God says you are. The truth is usually the opposite of the lie.

Take one of those lies and ask God who He says you are. Try to remember where and when you first thought that lie. Then picture Him coming in, and even what He would say and do, which is probably opposite of what you originally experienced.

Remember, He despised the shame so we wouldn't have to feel it.

---

[6] Neil T. Anderson, *Victory Over Darkness: Realize the Power of Your Identity in Christ* (Grand Rapids: Baker Books, 2010), 43.

[7] Michael Dye, *The Genesis Process for Change Groups, Book One* (Auburn: Michael Dye, 2006), 41.

✚ Write down all you saw and what He spoke to you.

_____

_____

_____

_____

_____

_____

✚ Now, ask God to give you a new picture. List the truth of who God says
you are on the new mirror that follows. Do the same for every lie you listed.

_____

_____

_____

_____

_____

_____

✚ After spending time with God to exchange the lie with a truth that God SHOWS
you (a right brain experience), find a logos word, whether on your own or
from this list, that validates what He has said.

_____

_____

_____

_____

_____

Who I Am In Christ

The Word of God says:

01. I am God's child for I am born again of the incorruptible seed of the Word of God that lives and abides forever. (1 Peter 1:23)

02. I am forgiven of all my sins and washed in the blood. (Ephesians 1:7; Hebrews 9:14; Colossians 1:14; 1 John 2:12; 1 John 1:9)

03. I am a new creation. (2 Corinthians 5:17)

04. I am a temple where the Holy Spirit lives. (1 Corinthians 6:19)

05. I am delivered from the power of darkness; Christ brings me into God's kingdom. (Colossians 1:13)

06. I am redeemed from the curse of the law. (1 Peter 1:18-19)

07. I am holy and without blame before God. (Ephesians 1:4)

08. I am established to the end. (1 Corinthians 1:8)

09. I am close to God - brought closer through the blood of Christ. (Ephesians 2:13)

10. I am victorious. (Revelation 21:7)

11. I am set free. (John 8:31-32)

12. I am strong in the Lord. (Ephesians 6:10)

13. I am dead to sin. (Romans 6:2 & 11; 1 Peter 2:24)

14. I am more than a conqueror. (Romans 8:37)

15. I am a co-heir with Christ. (Romans 8:16-17)

16. I am sealed with the Holy Spirit of promise. (Ephesians 1:13)

17. I am in Christ Jesus by His doing. (1 Corinthians 1:30)

18. I am accepted in Jesus Christ. (Ephesians 1:5-6)

19. I am complete in Him. (Colossians 2:10)

20. I am crucified with Christ. (Galatians 2:20)

21. I am alive with Christ. (Ephesians 2:4-5)

22. I am free from condemnation. (Romans 8:1)

23. I am reconciled to God. (2 Corinthians 5:18)

24. I am qualified to share in His inheritance. (Colossians 1:12)

25. I am firmly rooted, established in my faith and overflowing with gratefulness and thankfulness. (Colossians 2:7)

26. I am called by God. (2 Timothy 1:9)

27. I am chosen. (1 Thessalonians 1:4; Ephesians 1:4; 1 Peter 2:9)

28. I am an ambassador of Christ. (2 Corinthians 5:20)

29. I am God's workmanship created in Christ Jesus for good works. (Ephesians 2:10)

30. I am the apple of my Father's eye. (Deuteronomy 32:10; Psalm 17:8)

31. I am healed by the stripes of Jesus. (1 Peter 2:24; Isaiah 53:6)

32. I am being changed into His image. (2 Corinthians 3:18; Philippians 1:6)

33. I am raised up with Christ and am seated in heavenly places. (Ephesians 2:6)

34. I am God's beloved child. (Colossians 3:12; Romans 1:7; 1 Thessalonians 1:4)

35. I am sound of mind - with the mind of Christ. (Philippians 2:5; 1 Corinthians 2:16)

36. I am His heir and have obtained an inheritance. (Ephesians 1:11)

37. I am an overcomer because He has overcome the world. (1 John 5:4)

38. I am not condemned because I have everlasting life. (John 5:24; John 6:47)

39. I am a woman of peace covered with the peace of God that transcends all understanding. (Philippians 4:7)

40. I am a woman of power—with the power of the Holy Spirit indwelling me; power to lay hands on the sick and see them recover; power to cast out demons; power over all the power of the enemy; nothing shall by any means hurt me. (Mark 16:17-18; Luke 10:17-19)

41. I am indwelled by the Great One in me because greater is He who is in me than he who is in the world. (1 John 4:4)

42. I am always triumphant in Christ. (2 Corinthians 2:14)

43. I am hidden with Christ in God. (Colossians 3:3)

My *logos* word _____

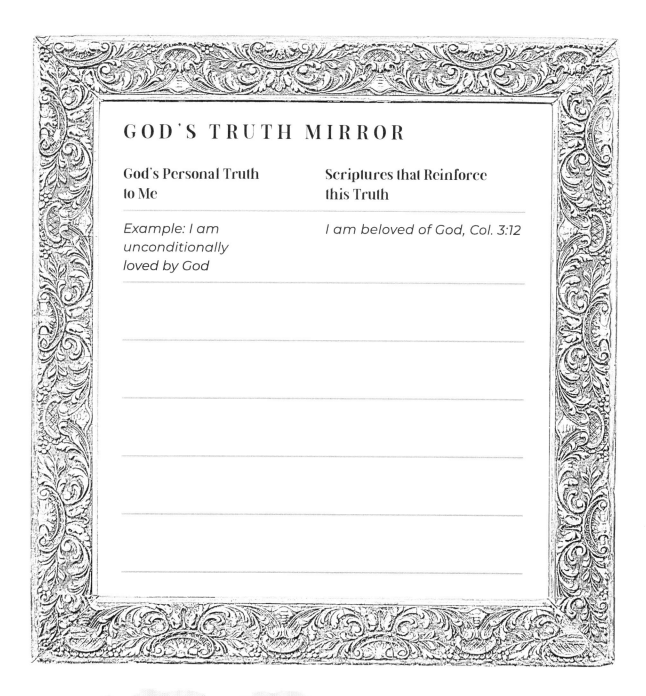

GOD'S TRUTH MIRROR

God's Personal Truth to Me	Scriptures that Reinforce this Truth
Example: I am unconditionally loved by God	*I am beloved of God, Col. 3:12*

✚ It may take a few weeks to hear God for all five lies. Spend time with God repeating this exercise until you have at least five personal promises (truths you've experienced) from God.

Commit to reviewing these truth Scriptures each day. This contributes to your healing. It helps to change your brain by filling your mind with what God has spoken to you, about you, based on how He sees you.

Living Beyond Betrayal

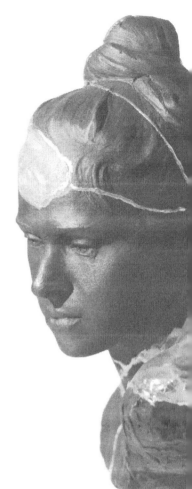

At this point, you may still have a lot of questions about the healing process. Many partners ask,

- Why do I need healing when I'm not the one with the problem?
- What does my emotional health have to do with my healing?
- How will discovering my personal promises from God help me heal from betrayal?
- Why do I need to be in a support group?
- When will I stop feeling triggered by his behaviors?

Many partners feel this way. They didn't ask for this. They're doing so much work to find healing, but still cannot shake the aftershocks of living beyond betrayal.

✚ **What questions do you still have about the healing process?**

_____

_____

_____

_____

_____

_____

_____

As I sat down to write my "goodbyes" to the man I had married, I remembered the song he wrote for me—a gift, full of hope and dreams. It said I had "shown him love and opened his heart, made his loneliness depart" and that "our love was growing, giving, molding us together day to day." It promised that God's love would "hold us, guide us, lead us in the everlasting way."

Yet here I am twenty-six years later...a lifetime away. Our life—shattered. Our love—destroyed. I never dreamed, imagined, or even thought divorce would ever happen to us. How could it? We both loved the Lord, served in ministry together, raised our family as believers, and led others to believe, too. Today, if I see a picture of him, I feel intense pain down deep into the core of my very being. It is a pain unlike any I have ever experienced in my life. It is fierce and violent, like parts of my being, deep inside, have been pressed into a huge shredder and are hanging, dripping with blood, still attached to me but not connected on the other end.

SHELBY

One of the greatest challenges for partners is picking up the pieces of our life—after it's been shattered by betrayal—and putting it back together. To some extent, we're creating something new. A new way of living in health and wholeness. And while this healing journey will take time, we can find comfort and hope in our heavenly Father.

> *You turned my wailing into dancing; you removed my sackcloth and clothed me with joy, that my heart may sing your praises and not be silent. LORD my God, I will praise you forever.*
>
> PSALM 30:11-12 (NIV)

The word "wailing" used here is a very different word for weeping. This word appears many times in the Bible and is often translated as lamenting or mourning. It is used to describe a response to great tragedy, death, or loss of relationship.

Teri: Like Shelby, since I experienced the shock and trauma of divorce as a consequence of my husband's sexual addiction, I was afraid to believe the promise this verse offered. I had experienced so many of my husband's broken promises like, "I will never _____ again" and "I will be faithful to you until death do us part," that I was afraid to even hope. But this verse has become one of my favorite promises in the Bible. It encouraged me to look at my "sackcloth" (loss and sadness) and allow myself to fully embrace and grieve my losses. And I have experienced it: God turned my mourning into dancing! He took away the anguish of being clothed in sadness and replaced it with gladness.

However, notice what God doesn't do. He doesn't simply stop our mourning and make it disappear. No, He transforms it...into joy! He turns our sorrow into gladness. He takes our loss and creates success! We serve an awesome and mighty God who says, *"All things work together for good to those who love Him, and to those who are called according to His purpose*" (Romans 8:28). **Our sorrows, disappointments, tragedies, and losses are very real, and they are also "raw material" for a divine transformation that our Lord will accomplish in His time, for His glory.** We WILL once again dance! Our part is to believe and cling to this wonderful promise!

✚ In what places of your life is it hardest to see God at work? Explain.

_____

_____

_____

_____

_____

_____

_____

_____

_____

_____

_____

_____

_____

_____

_____

_____

_____

✚ On the following chart, list some of the "raw materials" (e.g., sorrows, disappointments, tragedies, and losses) you would like God to transform for you.

In the second column, write down any transformation of those raw materials you might already see occurring in your life. You can come back to this page in the future to add how God has transformed your sorrow and pain into joy and dancing. I know He will do it for you because I have been privileged to see Him do it for me!

RAW MATERIALS	GOD'S TRANSFORMATION
Lost friendships due to discovery/disclosure	*New friends that understand the pain of betrayal; experiencing new, authentic, and real friendships.*

✚ Meditate on this Scripture and then share the positive things you see God doing even in the midst of your pain.

> You turned my wailing into dancing; you removed my sackcloth and clothed me with joy, that my heart may sing your praises and not be silent. LORD my God, I will praise you forever.
>
> PSALM 30:11-12 (NIV)

✚ In light of this Scripture and the raw materials chart you filled out, what could you expect God to do in the future?

_____

_____

_____

_____

_____

_____

_____

The Window of Tolerance

As we learn more about the healing process and understand the impact of betrayal trauma, it's important to recognize the effect it has on our emotional health and when we may be out of our "window of tolerance."[8] This model suggests that we all have an ability to navigate situations in our lives with appropriate emotional responses. This is our **"window"**—when we can face life's hurdles and emotionally tolerate our feelings without becoming emotionally dysregulated. However, on either side of our window there are two extremes: **hyperarousal**, when our sympathetic nervous system is activated (our fight, flight, or freeze response), or **hypoarousal**, when our parasympathetic nervous system is activated (fawn or fold response).

---

[8] Daniel J. Siegel, _The Developing Mind: How Relationships and the Brain Interact to Shape Who We Are_ (New York: The Guilford Press, 2020), 341-342.

As previously discussed, when we experience trauma, we may exhibit a plethora of physical and emotional responses. Sometimes, responses that don't even make sense to us in the moment. But understanding how trauma can decrease our window of tolerance may help to explain why we respond the way we do. The following table identifies some of the behaviors we might exhibit when we are in our window of tolerance and when we are outside our window.

Sympathetic-dominant Hyperarousal:

Emotionally flooded, reactive, impulsive, hypervigilant, fearful, angry.

Intrusive imagery and affects, racing thoughts

Flashbacks, nightmares, high-risk behavior

Efforts to reduce this state may include suicide planning, self harm, compulsive cleaning, abuse of alcohol or opiates

Freeze

Mute, terrified, frozen defense responses. High arousal coupled with physical immobility.

Window of Tolerance

Optimal arousal zone, encompassing both intense emotion and states of calm or relaxation, in which emotions can be tolerated and information integrated

Parasympathetic-dominant Hypoarousal:

Flat affect, numb, "empty" or "dead"

Cognitively dissociated, inability to think

Collapsed, disabled defensive responses

Helpless and hopeless

Efforts to reduce may include suicide planning, self-harm, compulsive

Table. Autonomic arousal in the wake of trauma: sympathetic hyperarousal and parasympathetic hypoarousal states drive emotional and autonomic dysregulation. Also shown is the frozen fear state in which both extremes may be present. States of optimal arousal and emotional regulation are relatively rare or difficult to maintain. Some examples are included of how dysfunctional behaviors can be utilized in the service of emotional regulation: both to reduce the intensity of the high arousal states and the depth of the low arousal states. Adapted from Ogden et al (2006) and Siegel (1999).[9]

[9] Frank Corrigan, J. Fisher, and David Nutt, "Autonomic dysregulation and the Window of Tolerance model of the effects of complex emotional trauma," Journal of Psychopharmacology, 25, January 2011, 17-25, doi:10.1177/0269881109354930.

✚ Which response do you identify with most, when you become more self-aware and recognize you are operating outside of your window of tolerance?

When we continue to live with untreated trauma—living in survival mode or as though our internal alarm is continuously signaling danger—our window of tolerance becomes more narrow. This creates more opportunity for us to be outside of our window rather than inside our window.

As a result of trauma, an individual may experience "...strong somatic responses in which the body tends to become frozen, collapsed or driven: action becomes either impossible or impulsive. Non-threatening situational cues often activate sympathetic nervous system (SNS) activity and fight–flight responses, while dangerous situations instead elicit parasympathetic non-responsiveness or submission– compliance responses."[10]

However, when we pursue healing and learn to navigate life's hurdles in a healthy way, we become more resilient and our window of tolerance gets wider. We become better equipped to tolerate and deal with stressful situations while maintaining our emotional response from within our window. In fact, as our window of tolerance expands, our hyperarousal and hypoarousal responses are minimized. When this happens, we know we are moving in the right direction toward lifelong health.

✚ When it comes to your window of tolerance, how well do you stay within your window? What type of situation creates hyperarousal or hypoarousal, where you move outside your window of tolerance? Explain.

[10] Corrigan, *Journal of Psychopharmacology*, 2011.

When we have been betrayed by someone we love and trust, we are thrust into a journey of painful loss and trauma. It is not a journey we chose, but a consequence we will live out because of the choices made by our spouse.

This is part of the human experience. Many of us will face various forms of pain, tragedy, trauma, and loss. And because of the unpredictable nature of loss, we may not know what's happening in our brain and body, or know what to do with it. A perfect example is given in the true story of Gerald Sittser:[11]

In the spring of 1996, Gerald Sittser and his family were traveling home from a mission trip when their car was hit head-on by a drunk driver. The crash changed his life. In that moment, he lost his wife, mother, and daughter. He was severely injured and he still had the responsibility of caring for his three other children. After he came home from the hospital he did not do well, even though he knew there was life before the trauma and there would be life after the trauma.

How do you cope with this kind of pain? Hear his words:

If normal, natural, reversible loss is like a broken limb, then catastrophic loss is like an amputation. The results are permanent, the impact incalculable, the consequences cumulative. Each new day forces one to face some devastating dimension of the loss. It creates a whole new context for one's life.[12]

Gerald began to have a recurring nightmare (which is a hyperarousal response to trauma and outside of his window of tolerance). In this nightmare he was walking on an endless beach with the sun low in the early evening sky. Darkness seemed to be gathering in the eastern sky and he feared being swallowed up in the darkness. Gerald began to run as fast as he could toward the setting sun hoping that he would be able to stay in the daylight. His nightmare ended in terror just as the sun set below the horizon and he was immersed in the darkness. Gerald woke up exhausted and drenched in perspiration after these nightmares because he had actually threshed in bed as he "ran" toward the setting sun.

He had this horrible nightmare every night for several weeks. This nightmare was consuming him whether he was awake or asleep. After several weeks, Gerald made a great choice. He called his sister and told her about his nightmare. She responded with an incredible and insightful comment.

She told him that nobody could catch the setting sun; she told him to turn, face the darkness and even run into the darkness, for in doing so, he would catch the rising sun.

---

[11] Gerald Sittser's story summarized by Harry Flanagan, *Seven Pillars of Freedom Workbook* (Gresham: Pure Desire Ministries International, 2009), 103-104.

[12] Gerald L. Sittser, *A Grace Disguised: How the Soul Grows Through Loss* (Grand Rapids: Zondervan, 2004), 32.

✚ As you reflect on your own pain and losses because of betrayal, how does this story of running into the darkness to catch the rising sun resonate with you? Explain.

_____

_____

_____

_____

_____

_____

_____

_____

✚ How does it give you hope for your future? Explain.

_____

_____

_____

_____

_____

_____

_____

_____

Note: If you are feeling triggered by any of the lesson content or this healing process, and want to pursue professional help, please contact Pure Desire at 503-489-0230 or visit **puredesire.org/counseling**; or contact APSATS (The Association of Partners of Sex Addicts Trauma Specialists) at 513-874-2342 or email **info@apsats.org**.

4

How Do I Keep Myself Safe and Sane While He Works His Recovery ?

Establishing Safety

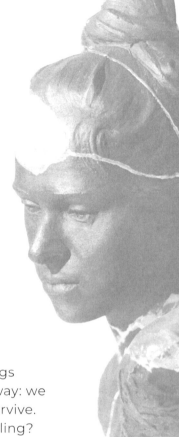

As we work through the next few lessons, we will be looking at the things we do to keep us safe. When in crisis, many of us have responded this way: we developed behaviors that protected us and kept us safe, so we could survive. But in the long run, are they helping us heal or interfering with our healing?

Sarah's story exemplifies behaviors that surfaced when attempting to navigate betrayal trauma and life in survival mode.

I need help! My husband is an out-of-control sex addict! I have known this for years and have done everything I can to help him break out of this. I look through every newspaper and magazine to make sure there are no pictures in it he might lust after. I even go in the bathroom while he showers to make sure he doesn't masturbate. Whenever we have errands, I pack up our disabled son to go with us because I can't trust him to go out alone and I can't leave him alone either. My grandmother needs surgery with three days of help afterward, but I'm afraid; if I go to help her, he may do something bad and won't be able to take care of our disabled son. Even though my parents are close by, I can't fully disclose to them what's happening; they already disapprove of my husband in so many ways.

I feel trapped in this marriage and am constantly on guard against his addiction. I don't know how much more he is doing, but he's never honest with me and we fight all the time. This is eating me alive and I'm a nervous wreck. Our finances are in shambles and we are a heartbeat away from bankruptcy. None of my friends seem to understand my issues and I feel so alone. As a Christian, I don't feel we should divorce, but we are in constant crisis! Help, I don't know what to do!

SARAH

✚ **What aspects of Sarah's story resonate with you? Explain.**

_____

_____

_____

_____

This story reflects the pain and anguish many women feel when trying to survive the complexity of betrayal trauma. They are attempting to recreate safety and doing their best to navigate this new, unstable reality.

Following discovery or disclosure, like Sarah, women often exert an enormous amount of energy into reestablishing healthy control in their environment so they feel safe.

Women naturally desire love, safety, nurturing relationships, and security. God made us this way. And yet, this natural predisposition and desire to protect ourselves can become harmful when we are motivated by fear. Sarah is caught in the trap of being fearful of relapse, feeling responsible for everyone, and only confident in herself to bring safety.

Sarah's story also illustrates how exhausted one can get, not only preoccupied with her husband's behavior, but keeping his secret from her family, and probably from her friends, too. She expended most of her energy helping the marriage get better, keeping tabs on her husband, and surviving as a mother. Sarah needed time to process her own painful trauma and find healthy solutions.

Her desire for truth and protection from further trauma may cause her to seek safety in ways that are not helpful in the long run. Realistically, she might be feeling hopeless and insecure about her own future. All of these stress factors contribute to safety-seeking behaviors. Sometimes to the point where a betrayed partner is neglecting her own needs.

✚ **In what ways have you neglected your own needs because of the stress brought on by betrayal? Explain.**

_____

_____

_____

_____

_____

✚ **What effect is this neglect having on you: emotionally, physically, and spiritually ?**

When it comes to making our needs a priority, our thoughts may immediately go to Scriptures that say, as Christians, we should give to anyone who asks (Matthew 5:42). If you read the context of this Scripture, Jesus is describing a radically selfless behavior. There is another Scripture that speaks to putting the needs of others above our own needs.

> *Do nothing out of selfish ambition or vain conceit. Rather, in humility value others above yourselves, not looking to your own interests but each of you to the interests of the others.*
>
> PHILIPPIANS 2:3-4 (NIV)

This is not saying to neglect our needs, but to also consider the needs of others. Not because others are more important than us, but because it's describing what a healthy relationship looks like: where the needs of both people in the relationship are taken into consideration.

Scripture also says to love your neighbor as yourself (Mark 12:31). It is difficult to fully love others, if you are not loving and taking care of yourself. The Apostle Paul shares some significant guidelines for healthy relationships which we will develop further in Lesson 2 when we talk about healthy boundaries.

> ***Carry each other's burdens***, *and in this way you will fulfill the law of Christ...Each one should test their own actions. Then they can take pride in themselves alone, without comparing themselves to someone else,* ***for each one should carry their own load****.*
>
> GALATIANS 6:2, 4-5 (NIV, EMPHASIS ADDED)

In verse 2, the Greek term "burden" refers to a very heavy load that could be crushing for one person to carry alone. In verse 5, the term "load" refers to a manageable bundle a person could carry on their back. Paul contrasts the difference for believers so they would know how to handle difficulties in relationships. He states we must each take responsibility for ourselves and when our burden is too great, others can come in and help us to lighten the impact. Likewise, you can also bless others by sharing their burdens when they are overloaded, while still shouldering your own responsibilities. This interdependence fulfills "the law of Christ."[1]

A pastor friend, Cliff Hanes, shared a story that helped me picture the difference. Cliff was invited by his brother to go on a mountain climbing adventure. His brother, who was an experienced climber, gave Cliff a list of the things he needed to carry up the mountain in his backpack. Cliff's inexperience and apprehensions came to the surface as he complained to his brother that carrying forty pounds as a novice mountain climber was going to be difficult. His brother said, "If you want to go on this adventure, you need to carry your own load." This pack included Cliff's sleeping bag, food, layers of clothing, personal climbing equipment, and toiletries. Cliff's brother went on to explain that he himself was carrying seventy-five pounds. This not only included what he needed personally, but it also included cooking utensils, a tent, lantern, and extra equipment they both needed for the climb. Since this was Cliff's first climb, his brother only expected Cliff to carry his own load. Cliff's brother was willing to carry the extra burden for the adventure to be a success.

In life, God will give us people like this brother who realize we can't shoulder our burdens alone. Your leader and those in your group can help shoulder your burden. But there are some things only you can carry. The great relief comes when we realize we are not traveling alone on this journey and all of us have to carry something.

The problem comes when people don't carry their own load—what is their own responsibility. To compound the problem, there is a lot of confusion about respecting, defining, and maintaining personal boundaries in relationships. Often, the addict is so consumed with his sexual behaviors that he ignores carrying his appropriate load: using manipulation, gaslighting, guilt, and shame to coerce others into carrying his load. Without fully understanding the impact of their actions, some partners may end up carrying the load of their spouse because they've been told it's their wifely duty or maybe out of fear that something bad will happen if they don't cover for the addict.

In order for your husband to find lifelong recovery and healing, he needs to take responsibility for his behaviors and **experience the natural consequences of his actions.** When the law of sowing and reaping is upheld, "the natural consequences are falling on the shoulders of the responsible party."[2] It sounds so well intentioned when a partner takes on extra responsibility; however, it often delays the healing process for her and her husband.

---

[1] Henry Cloud and John Townsend, Boundaries: *When to Say YES. When to Say NO, to Take Control of Your Life* (Grand Rapids: Zondervan, 1992), 30.

[2] Cloud and Townsend, *Boundaries*, 156.

Consider Sarah's story at the beginning of this lesson. Look at the responsibility she has taken on: keeping her husband sober, protecting his reputation with her family, caring for her extended family member in addition to her special needs child, and fearing financial ruin. God never designed her to carry the weight of the marriage, fix her husband, or hold together their family and extended family.

✚ **If Sarah was your friend, how would you encourage her to make her healing a priority? What suggestions or strategies would you recommend for her to start taking care of her needs?**

As we get to know ourselves, understand how trauma has impacted us, and how it contributes to why we do what we do, we become better equipped to take care of ourselves. And this happens best when we make our healing a priority.

✚ Use the following table to identify specific needs that you have been neglecting. Then identify one thing you can do to meet the need and the first step you can take to make it happen. A couple examples are listed to get you started.

A Need I've Been Neglecting	One Thing I Can Do To Meet This Need	First Step
I've been neglecting time to myself or time to do what I want to do.	Create time and space in my schedule to have time to myself and/or focus on what I want to do.	I will talk with my husband about creating time for myself in the evenings, so he can watch the kids. I'll also talk with my mom about watching the kids one morning each week, so I can take an art class.
I've been neglecting my physical health.	I'm going to start working out 4 days a week.	I'm going to join a gym near my house. My friend and I will work out together to keep each other accountable.

Having the support of safe people is a foundational part of healing from betrayal. But after living with a person who regularly lied and manipulated you, it may be tough to identify who is a safe person and who is not.

In the book, *Safe People*, authors Cloud and Townsend state that someone with healthy boundaries and a good sense of self-assertiveness usually won't have to leave the relationship. Instead, the addict will feel so uncomfortable with the new boundaries and knowing these boundaries will be reinforced, that he will either change or be the one who leaves the relationship.[3]

For many partners, what should concern them most is the attitude of her husband's heart. The following list helps women determine what that heart looks like.

✚ **Look at the following characteristics of safe and unsafe people:[4]**

SAFE PEOPLE	UNSAFE PEOPLE
• Admit their weaknesses	• Think they "have it all together"
• Are spiritual	• Are religious
• Are open to feedback	• Are defensive
• Are humble	• Are self-righteous
• Apologize and change behavior	• Only apologize
• Deal with the problems	• Avoid working on their problems
• Earn trust	• Demand trust
• Admit their faults	• Believe they are perfect
• Take responsibility	• Blame others
• Tell the truth	• Lie
• Are growing	• Are stagnant

✚ **In your life right now, who would you consider safe people? Make a list using first names or initials.**

• _____   • _____

• _____   • _____

• _____   • _____

• _____   • _____

---

[3] Henry Cloud and John Townsend, *Safe People: How to Find Relationships that are Good for You and Avoid Those that Aren't* (Grand Rapids: Zondervan, 1995), 189-199.

[4] Cloud and Townsend, *Safe People*, 27-38.

✚ What is it that makes them a safe person?

_____

_____

_____

_____

_____

✚ After reading this list, can you identify areas where your husband may seem unsafe? Explain.

_____

_____

_____

_____

_____

✚ In light of what you have learned about establishing safety and safe people, write a prayer for yourself asking God for wisdom and discernment in this area of your healing.

_____

_____

_____

_____

_____

Establishing Healthy Boundaries

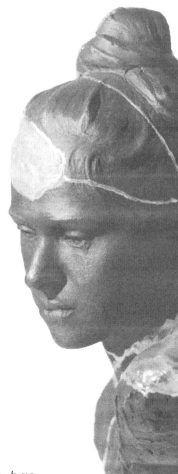

I have grown children who are now out of the home. My husband, Dave, has served time in jail for having been inappropriate with minors but is soon to be released. He says he made a commitment to Christ while incarcerated, but I haven't seen it impact or change his walk. I am not sure if our marriage will survive but he wants to stay with me because as a convicted felon, it will be hard for him to find another place to stay. Dave has told me that as a Christian, Jesus would expect me to forgive and start repairing the marriage.

My children are outraged that I would even consider that kind of arrangement. Although they have not personally expressed any sexual abuse by him, they are concerned for their children (our grandchildren). I feel torn; I still love him and really don't want to live the rest of my life alone. I also love my children who are considering cutting ties with me if I allow him back. They think I am wanting to rescue him. What should I do?

DONNA

✚ **How would you respond to Donna's dilemma? What advice would you give her?**

_____

_____

_____

_____

_____

_____

How do we learn to navigate relationships in a way that is safe and healthy? The first step is learning how to set and walk in healthy boundaries.

Donna was faced with a difficult decision. Her adult children were out of the home and very alarmed that Mom would even consider such an arrangement. In counseling her, I told her that her children had every right to feel the way they did because they had also been betrayed and had suffered many consequences (shame, abandonment, financial struggles, and having to be raised by a single mom). It was important for her to validate her children's feelings and to acknowledge that she, too, had concerns.

In the end, it would be her choice as to what she wanted to do. Ultimately, she was the one who had to live with the consequences. If she was willing to give her husband a second chance, she would have to do it with strong determination, which included these steps:

- Think through reasonable consequences and if ignored, seek wise counsel.

- Write a Safety Action Plan that includes the boundaries and natural consequences if he violates those boundaries.

- Establish a group of women who are willing to support her with prayer and encourage her to follow through with her Safety Action Plan.

- Validate her children's feelings and share her own concerns. Show them her Safety Action Plan and the natural consequences if there are any boundary violations.

- Ask them what their boundaries are for her with respect to the grandchildren (e.g., Does she need to come to their homes to see them? Should she require her husband to leave her home while the grandchildren are visiting?) Whatever they request would be part of her Safety Action Plan with which he would have to comply.

These were some of the healthy boundaries Donna included in her Safety Action Plan.

Where are you when it comes to boundaries? How hard is it for you to set healthy boundaries? The following questions will help you think through what your present behaviors look like when it comes to boundaries.

✚ On a scale of 1-10 (ten being very difficult), how difficult is it for you to feel like a loving person and set healthy boundaries at the same time? Circle one.

1	2	3	4	5	6	7	8	9	10

Not Difficult   Very Difficult

✚ In a sentence or two, describe what you think is a real boundary.

_____

_____

_____

_____

✚ What do you think and feel if someone is upset because of a boundary you have set (e.g., spouse, relative, or close friend)?

_____

_____

_____

_____

_____

✚ How do you respond when faced with someone else's boundaries? Explain.

_____

_____

_____

_____

_____

What does Jesus and the Bible say about boundaries?

Being married to an addict can create challenges to living out a healthy relationship. This is why it is important to have a biblical perspective on what Jesus says about boundaries. The book *Boundaries* gives us a great biblical definition of what boundaries are and are not.

In short, boundaries are not walls. The Bible does not say that we are to be "walled off" from others; in fact, it says that we are to be one with them (John 17:11). We are to be in community with them. But in every community, all members have their own space and property. The important thing is that property lines are permeable enough to allow passing and strong enough to keep out danger. Often, when people are abused while growing up, they reverse the function of boundaries and keep the bad in and the good out.[5]

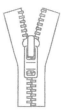 One of the best pictures illustrating healthy boundaries versus shame-based boundaries is illustrated with a zipper metaphor in the book, *Facing the Shame*.[6] The authors explain how shame-based people have zippers on the outside of their lives and anyone can have access to those zippers. Healthy people have zippers on the inside of their lives and they control who has access.

Revelation 3:20 (NASB) shows that Jesus respects our boundaries:

> *Behold, I stand at the door and knock; if anyone hears My voice and opens the door, I will come in to him and will dine with him, and he with Me.*
>
> REVELATION 3:20 (NASB)

Maybe you have seen this concept beautifully illustrated in the picture of Jesus knocking at a door that has no knob on the outside because the door can only be opened from the inside. God has given us control over our relationship with Him. We choose when to let Him in and how much we want to yield to Him.

God has also designed us for relationship with others, and He desires that we have healthy boundaries in place. As stated in the previous definition, boundaries are not designed to keep people out. In fact, **those who have appropriate boundaries actually increase their ability to care about others.**

Jesus was the most compassionate and caring person that ever lived. Yet, Jesus had

---

[5] Henry Cloud and John Townsend, *Boundaries: When to Say YES. When to Say NO, to Take Control of Your Life* (Grand Rapids: Zondervan, 1992), 32.

[6] Merie A. Fossum and Marilyn J. Mason, *Facing Shame: Families in Recovery* (New York: W.W. Norton & Co., 1989), 70-71.

healthy boundaries in place that released Him to care effectively for people. Let's look at some Scriptures from the Gospel of Mark (NIV) that repeatedly show how Jesus set boundaries to take care of His own needs and those of His twelve disciples.

> *The whole town gathered at the door...Jesus healed many...Very early in the morning...Jesus got up, left the house and went off to a solitary place...and when they found him, they exclaimed: "Everyone is looking for you!" ...Jesus could no longer enter a town openly but stayed outside in lonely places.*
>
> MARK 1:33-37, 45 (NIV)

✝ **What do these verses tell us about Jesus' boundaries?**

_____

_____

_____

_____

_____

> *...[He] called to him those he wanted...He appointed twelve... (Mark 3:13-14)*
>
> *...the man...begged to go with him. Jesus did not let him... (Mark 5:18-19)*
>
> *...He did not let anyone follow him except... (Mark 5:37)*
>
> *...Jesus did not want anyone to know where they were, because he was teaching his disciples. (Mark 9:30-31)*

✝ **These Scriptures clearly show Jesus' decision to limit and/or give access to people. What are the implications for our lives?**

_____

_____

_____

_____

...he told his disciples to have a small boat ready for him, to keep the people from crowding him. (Mark 3:9)

✚ **What does this Scripture imply about the balance of having friends help us when we need it?**

_____

_____

_____

Notice that in caring for others, Jesus also recognized His need to care for Himself. He withdrew and even said "no" in order to be effective and remain healthy. He made requests and did not meet every demand made of Him. In fact, when Jesus became the sacrifice for our sins, He made it clear it was His decision.[7]

> *For this reason the Father loves Me, because I lay down My life so that I may take it again. No one has taken it away from Me, but I lay it down on My own initiative..*
>
> JOHN 10:17-18A (NASB1995)

When we don't have much experience with it, setting healthy boundaries can be challenging and may impact several areas of our life.

For many partners, because we were continually manipulated and lied to by our spouse, we may not have recognized when we allowed others to set our boundaries for us. Also, many Christian women were taught that serving in church is our responsibility. So saying "no" wasn't really an option.

✚ **Share about a time you relinquished your boundary and allowed someone else to set a boundary for you.**

_____

_____

_____

_____

_____

---

[7] Byron Kehler, concept from "Self-Care" Handout (Milwaukie: Agape Youth & Family Ministries, 1992).

✚ Share about a time when you reluctantly said "yes" to something or committed to something you later regretted.

_____
_____
_____
_____
_____
_____

✚ What is your greatest challenge in setting healthy boundaries?

_____
_____
_____
_____
_____
_____

✚ What experiences might have caused you to think that the zipper in your life needed to be on the outside, giving anyone and everyone access? Explain.

_____
_____
_____
_____
_____
_____

For many partners, setting boundaries is a huge step in their healing. Communicating a boundary can sometimes take a bit of finesse and practice. Here's a great formula to use: When you...I feel...I need...if you can't do this, I will...[8] Here's what communicating a boundary might look like:

When you take your phone to bed, **I feel** unsafe and fear you will act out again. **I need** to see you act in ways that protect us. **If you** keep taking your phone to bed with you, **I will** ask you to sleep in another room (or ask you to put your phone elsewhere). **If you** aren't willing to do this, **I will** no longer sleep with you (or no longer keep this a secret from our friends or consider what I need to do to protect myself).

A boundary violation results in the betrayed partner taking action of some kind to protect herself or to act in ways that reflect reality.

✚ Let's put this into practice: think of a recent time where you put a boundary in place. Now use this formula to write out how you might communicate this boundary.

- When you _____
- I feel _____
- I need _____
- If you can't do this, I will _____

Learning this skill of communicating boundaries will be essential to your healing and empower you to take healthy control over the amount of access people have in your life.

✚ Make a list of people who have had too much access to your life and what the repercussions or consequences were for you.

Name of Person	Repercussions/consequences

[8] Barbara Steffens, Consultation, September 2022.

✚ Make a list of people with whom you have seen good boundaries.
Next to each person's name, write down how their good boundaries
affected you and your relationship.

Name of Person   Effect on You/the Relationship

_____

_____

_____

_____

✚ Of those traits you observed in others, list two or three you would like
to incorporate into your life. Explain how you plan to do this more.
Check the one you would like to work on this week.

_____

_____

_____

_____

✚ Since learning to set healthy boundaries is such an important step
to your healing, write out a prayer asking God to open your heart and mind
to begin to see boundaries from His perspective. Let Him know you are
willing to make healthy changes in this area.

_____

_____

_____

_____

As we pursue healing and learn to set healthy boundaries, we will also need to recognize when our boundaries are being violated. Boundary violations may not be obvious to us because we lived with an addict, which created an environment that was traumatic.

The following Abuse Inventory from Doug Weiss' book, *Partners: Healing From His Addiction*,[9] will help you identify boundary violations.

✚ **Check the statements that you have experienced in your relationship with the sex addict.**

Abuse Inventory

From *Partners: Healing From His Addiction* by Doug Weiss

Physical Violations:

☐ Somebody invading your "space"

☐ Being touched in ways that might make you feel uncomfortable, without first being asked

☐ Being told what you can or cannot wear for clothing or regarding the use of makeup

☐ Not having freedom to go as you please

☐ Being pushed, shoved, slapped, bitten, kicked, hit, punched, or choked

☐ Being tickled without permission

☐ Being threatened with a weapon

☐ Being forced to stay awake

☐ Being raped

☐ Other _____

Emotional Violations:

☐ Being told "You shouldn't feel that way"

☐ Having your expressed feelings ignored

☐ Being exposed to uncontrolled anger

☐ Being threatened with abandonment or forced to leave

---

[9] Doug Weiss, *Partners: Healing From His Addiction* (Colorado Springs: Discovery Press, 2001), 74-77.

- ☐ Being called names
- ☐ Having affections withheld
- ☐ Being told you are responsible for someone else's feelings (e.g. "You make me angry/sad/ embarrassed!")
- ☐ Not being allowed to cry or being forced to stuff your feelings out of fear
- ☐ Other _____

Spiritual Violations:

- ☐ The quoting of Scripture to force you to change
- ☐ Having your relationship with God decided for you
- ☐ Manipulation using God's authority
- ☐ Keeping you from church/church people
- ☐ Other _____

Intellectual Violations:

- ☐ Being told you are crazy or stupid
- ☐ Having your ability to reason things out for yourself discounted
- ☐ Not being allowed to go back to school or work
- ☐ Being blamed for your children's failures
- ☐ Having your parenting abilities discounted
- ☐ Not being allowed to make everyday choices
- ☐ Having words put in your mouth or twisted to infer things you didn't say
- ☐ Other _____

Financial Violations:

- ☐ Not being allowed to earn or spend your own money
- ☐ Struggling to pay for necessities when the addict spent money on porn or acting-out behavior
- ☐ Allowing the addict to take money from you to support his habit
- ☐ Being forced to account for every cent you spend
- ☐ Allowing the addict's spending to interfere with your family's welfare or health
- ☐ Being lied to about finances
- ☐ Other _____

Sexual Violations:

- ☐ Not respecting your right to say "no" to sex
- ☐ Touching you sexually without permission
- ☐ Treating you as a sex object
- ☐ Criticizing you sexually
- ☐ Withholding affection for sex
- ☐ Exposing you to pornography
- ☐ Insisting you wear clothing that you find inappropriate
- ☐ Expressing interest in other women while you are with him
- ☐ Sexualizing affectionate touch from you
- ☐ Making unsolicited comments about your body
- ☐ Demanding sex or certain types of sexual acts
- ☐ Minimizing or ignoring your feelings about sex
- ☐ Having affairs outside your marriage
- ☐ Exposing you to sexually transmitted diseases
- ☐ Making sexual jokes
- ☐ Buying clothing for you that you are uncomfortable wearing (the gift is really for him)
- ☐ Being physically forced or threatened with harm if you don't perform certain sexual acts
- ☐ Other _____

✚ **What is your response to the number of violations you checked? Explain.**

_____

_____

_____

_____

_____

_____

_____

If you made checks in several of the categories, remember: violations become commonplace when we live without healthy boundaries.

My Safety Action Plan

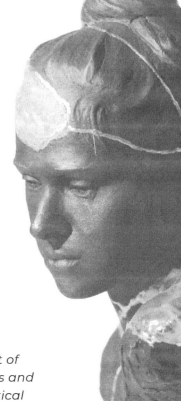

I need help in knowing how to proceed. My husband of 20 years is totally out of control regarding his sexual addiction. He has been visiting massage parlors and seeing prostitutes and squandering our money, all the while being hypercritical of other Christians' lives. He has used force and physical intimidation against me recently, but his fierce anger and cruel emotional manipulation have been growing for years, justified by him because he says I will not meet his sexual "needs" willingly or gladly. I have tried for years to confront him as a godly, submissive wife, but have been accused of the opposite, usually with name-calling, disgust, or Scripture thrown back in my face. On the one hand, I can see how wrong he is for these behaviors, but on the other hand, I hear condemnation for myself because I must be the problem.

Through the years various pieces of the sexual addiction would surface; somehow I thought that because of his repentance and "integrity" we would be able to work on these issues by ourselves. We had, after all, come a long way from our families that included addicts, controllers, and trauma. Additionally, he's been in a men's accountability group and has connections to well-known men in Christian circles. I've tried to trust him as a leader in our home, but he has used anger as a weapon and I have withdrawn more and more to just survive.

I can see now that I have essentially been shutting down for years amidst the shame and futile attempts to please him. I have lost myself in the process. I no longer have a life, my own friends, or my own passions. I don't even know who I am anymore. I have been able to take a month away from him and have slowly been seeing clearly for the first time what the issues were from the beginning of our marriage. I'm really struggling with boundaries, with how to state things properly so it doesn't enrage him, and with finding my own identity in the midst of this crisis. I'm not sure how to go forward, but I know I can't go backward.

DANAE

✚ **In light of what you've learned so far about the effects of trauma, list the symptoms of trauma and/or trauma responses you see in Danae's behaviors.**

_____

_____

_____

_____

_____

_____

In the previous lessons we looked at what the Bible says about boundaries and evaluated where we are with establishing healthy boundaries for ourselves. Differentiating between our responsibility and the other person's responsibility is often difficult when we feel unsafe in a relationship due to a spouse's addictive behaviors and betrayal.

So how do we establish healthy boundaries after betrayal? These three questions are important to ask yourself:

01. What is the desired outcome I seek?

02. For whom is the boundary intended?

03. Am I protecting myself or trying to change the addict?

In the opening story, Danae was faced with a difficult decision. Her husband had been visiting massage parlors, seeing prostitutes, and squandering their money. He used force and physical intimidation against her, was fiercely angry and emotionally manipulative, blamed his sex addition on her for not meeting his "needs," and was verbally and spiritually abusive. He had been in a men's accountability group and had connections with well-known men in Christian circles.

They had been separated for a month when Danae stated, "I'm really struggling with boundaries, with how to state things properly so it doesn't enrage him, and with finding my own identity in the midst of this crisis. I'm not sure how to go forward, but I know I can't go backward."

For Danae to move forward, she had some choices to make. If she was willing to reconcile with her husband, she would need a strong plan and support with completing these steps:

- Think through what it looks like to establish healthy boundaries in their relationship and what she needs to feel safe.

- Identify reasonable consequences specific to each type of boundary violation: physical, emotional, spiritual, sexual, and financial.
- Write a Safety Action Plan that includes the boundaries and consequences if her husband violates these boundaries.
- Establish a group of women who are willing to support her with prayer and help her follow through with her Safety Action Plan.

We went through the list of questions stated at the beginning of this lesson regarding motivation. This is the summary of her responses:

What is the desired outcome I seek in setting boundaries? Danae wanted to give him a second chance to rebuild trust in their relationship. The boundaries weren't there to control his behaviors; they were in place because she wanted to feel safe and be able to rebuild trust in him.

For whom is the boundary intended? Am I protecting myself or am I trying to change the addict? I tried to help her see that if she puts boundaries in place to change him, it would not work. But if she decides ahead of time what she needs to feel safe, she can share with him her Safety Action Plan and he can choose to follow the plan to earn trust or he can choose to leave the relationship. This gives him the opportunity to choose and experience the consequences of the betrayal and mistrust he has sown in the marriage.

Based on her situation, these were a few key aspects to Danae's Safety Action Plan. She would ask her husband to:

- Commit to professional counseling together, with a counselor who specializes in sex addiction and betrayal trauma, who can help with anger and abuse issues.
- Attend a weekly Pure Desire men's group and connect with the other men at least three times a week for accountability.
- Attend a domestic abuser's group to get his anger under control.
- Complete The FASTER Scale each week and share this with his accountability partner.
- Take a polygraph every three months for the first year and possibly less the following year. (See the appendix, page 326 for more information about the polygraph.)

If he agrees to her Safety Action Plan, there is a possibility for healing the marriage. If he refuses, he, in essence, is saying that he doesn't want to do whatever it would take to restore trust and save the marriage.

After writing this out, I asked her, "Can you live with the possibility that he may refuse and your marriage may end because he is unwilling to do the hard things restoration requires?" It was one of the most difficult choices she had ever made and she agreed this was the only hope for her marriage.

After creating her full Safety Action Plan, she shared it with the women in her support group. It is one thing to create a Safety Action Plan; it is another thing to follow through when the addict tries to manipulate or minimize what he has agreed to do. **Compliance for him and following through for her will be the most difficult behaviors they will need to learn.** The addict has spent his life manipulating to keep his addiction going. Danae, in various ways, has been stuck in survival mode, unable to make healthy choices for herself and for the relationship.

Although you may not see the importance of this task right now, most women have reported that this exercise of writing out and following through with consequences was the defining moment that helped their marriage move in a new direction. The leaders of Pure Desire men's groups have also reported that the men whose wives have a Safety Action Plan have fewer relapses and are more committed to do the hard work it takes to walk in health and wholeness.

Safety Action Plan

Note: *a Safety Action Plan is created by a betrayed partner; a Recovery Action Plan is created by the addicted spouse. While they are identical in some ways, each is unique to the individual and their situation, with a specific focus on either healing from betrayal or recovery from compulsive sexual behaviors. The content covered in this lesson is specific to a betrayed partner and what she needs to feel safe and rebuild trust in the relationship.*

The Safety Action Plan is a valuable tool for betrayed partners who want to take a proactive approach to healing their relationship.

Your Safety Action Plan will be a resource you can use to identify reasonable and necessary steps to take in response to a relapse by your spouse. Before joining a Pure Desire group, sexual acting out was a way of medicating pain. Now, as your spouse learns to walk in sobriety, your Safety Action Plan will give you and your spouse a new tool to help transform compulsive sexual behaviors and an appropriate response to those behaviors in your marriage.

The goal is to reestablish trust and implement actions that need to be taken in order to process the relapse and trauma in a proactive, intentional manner. This approach encourages the partner—and the spouse, when possible—to identify natural and logical consequences if a relapse occurs. Natural consequences are the inevitable result of the addict's own actions. Logical consequences happen as a result of the addict's actions, but are imposed by the partner or the addict themselves.

These consequences are not meant to be punitive. Rather, they are designed to help you, as a partner:

01. feel safe and learn to respond, rather than react to a relapse;

02. recognize WHERE your spouse is taking concrete steps toward recovery; and

03. rebuild trust in your marriage.

Keep in mind: develop a Safety Action Plan **for yourself.** If your spouse gets to the point in recovery where they have created their own Recovery Action Plan, combine your Safety/Recovery Action Plans. Schedule a good time to talk, when you both share your plan with each other in a non-reactive way. Communicating your Safety Action Plan to your spouse will help you find your voice and share honestly how your spouse's behavior affects you.

FOR GROUP MEMBERS WHO ARE SEPARATED OR DIVORCED

Your Safety Action Plan will provide additional boundaries and direction in dealing with coparenting, as well as establishing individual and relational health, regardless of the marriage outcome. Healing family system issues that involve sexual addiction can be painful, emotional, and especially challenging if the children have two separate homes. It is important to have clarity, support, and well defined goals that are specific to managing a separation or divorce in a way that reduces the impact this trauma may have on you and your children.

If your situation has escalated to the point where separation or divorce is necessary, your boundaries and healing steps will also need to be redefined, according to what the relationship is now and the desired outcome: reconciliation or divorce and coparenting, with as little damage as possible. If your divorce is final, and you are experiencing stability and healthy boundaries, then you may choose to use the Three Circles Exercise instead of a Safety Action Plan.

Everyone who completes a Safety Action Plan should find trusted individuals to share their plan with: your group members would be the ideal place to start.

> *Plans fail for lack of counsel, but with many advisers they succeed!*
>
> PROVERBS 15:22 (NIV)

CONSEQUENCES

When an addict can start associating their actions with a specific consequence, it will help them weigh the outcome of their behavior and whether it's worth the risk. The pain of consequences also creates change in the punishment/reward center of the brain. If the brain begins to connect painful consequences to a relapse, a person is less likely to choose that path. Consequences help an addict own the effects of their behavior rather than withdrawing, blaming, hiding, lying, getting angry, or spiraling down into the depths of shame. **Consequences will help you respond to your spouse's relapse in a non-reactive way.**

Predetermined consequences, which have been discussed with wise counsel, will empower you to make healthy decisions for yourself and feel safe in the situation. As painful as relapse is, having consequences decided ahead of time will allow you to fall back on your plan instead of allowing your emotions to take the wheel. After a relapse occurs, it may be tempting to bring peace to your relationship or yourself as quickly as possible. This approach is not effective for long-term health and healing. Having consequences written out ahead of time will give you the ability to immediately take action without falling back into old behaviors of "trying to make this all go away."

NATURAL CONSEQUENCES VS. LOGICAL CONSEQUENCES

Natural Consequences

A natural consequence occurs as a result of a choice, without anyone imposing it. Here are some examples of natural consequences for when your husband relapses:

- Trust is broken, and I feel betrayed when my husband acts out sexually. I feel hurt, a lack of safety, and alone.

- A relapse creates guilt or shame in my husband, which makes him withdraw and pull away from me.

- My husband's addiction costs valuable time, energy, and money that could have been invested in our relationship and family.

Logical Consequences

A logical consequence is a reasonable and necessary outcome imposed personally or by another. These are examples of logical consequences your husband might face after a relapse:

- Since he acted out after watching YouTube videos alone late at night, I will ask him to turn off all electronics after 10:30 pm and disable access to YouTube.

- His cell phone continues to be a source for viewing inappropriate images, so I will ask him to disable the Internet through our phone carrier.

- When on social media, he has flirted with others. I will ask him to close his account or only have a joint account with me.

Identify behaviors or actions that would help you see your spouse's sincerity and commitment to the marriage. The Safety Action Plan is designed to give you a clear picture of what you need in order to process the pain and feel free enough to move forward in your healing process. Essentially, you are creating a detailed list of actions your spouse can take in order to reestablish and regain trust in the relationship. Rebuilding trust takes intentionality and time.

Step 1: Identify what constitutes a relapse in your mind. When has your spouse crossed a line that requires intentional recovery? The goal is not to make your spouse perfect in every way, but to identify which behaviors, specifically, cause a fracture in your trust and relationship.

Step 2: Determine who your spouse needs to share their relapse with, and in what time frame. This typically includes a group member, a mentor or friend, and you. A good time frame is to share within 24 hours of the relapse.

Step 3: Write out natural consequences of your spouse's behavior. Some examples are noted at the end of this lesson. Try to be clear about how their behavior impacts you.

Step 4: Write out logical consequences connected to the behavior that would help you see that your spouse recognizes the serious nature of their actions. Again, some examples are listed at the end of this lesson.

Step 5: Make a list of steps you will need to personally take in order to feel safe and regain stability, in preparation to fully engage in the relationship. Examples are given at the end of this lesson.

Step 6: Describe your desired outcome for creating this plan. If you have a clear vision of how this plan will help you rebuild trust, you are more likely to follow it. The goal of a Safety Action Plan is not punitive, but to keep you focused on what steps are needed to rebuild trust.

If a relapse occurs, review your written Safety Action Plan and begin to implement it immediately. When lying, manipulating, blaming, hiding, and withdrawal take place after a relapse, it will only make recovery more difficult and increase the likelihood of multiple relapses. In order to encourage your spouse to come clean right away, consequences should be greater if the relapse isn't disclosed within 24 hours. Again, having measurable consequences is the key.

REBUILDING TRUST

Rebuilding trust takes intentionality and time. When trust is broken, it can be a long rebuilding process. It will be important for your spouse to be patient in reestablishing trust, even while actively working on the relationship. Before full disclosure, there were probably many lies and deceptions present in your marriage. Because of this, it will be difficult for you to trust your spouse's words or your own instinct. You will need to SEE behaviors that will help you start trusting again. You're learning how to believe behaviors and not just words. Your spouse's willingness to do the things necessary for you to feel safe enough to trust again is going to be the key to your marital health and reconciliation.

You are encouraged to identify behaviors or actions that would help you recognize your spouse is sincere and committed to the marriage. The Safety Action Plan is meant to give your spouse a clear picture of **what you need** in order to process your pain and feel free enough to move forward in the relationship. Essentially, you are giving your spouse a detailed list of things they can do in order to regain trust. When your spouse shows that they are absolutely committed to following this plan, even without your insistence or pressure, they will begin building trust after a relapse.

The Safety Action Plan is an outline that provides examples of what may be included in a plan. Additional action steps, or behaviors, may be incorporated to best meet the needs of those involved. When stuck or uncertain about how to proceed, consult with your group leader, other group members, or counselor.

YOUR PERSONAL SAFETY ACTION PLAN

Use the following space to begin creating your personal Safety Action Plan. If you need help, your leader and the women in your group may have ideas and suggestions. Also, there are several examples and action steps listed at the end of this lesson for you to reference if needed. This may help to give you a balanced perspective when creating your Safety Action Plan.

The first step is very important because it says to your husband you are committed to the process. With the second step, try and choose only the things you need right now for your spouse to commit to. Many of the options may not reflect where your relationship is at this point.

It is recommended that you review your plan every six months and eliminate those items or action steps that no longer apply and add new ones (i.e. a marriage seminar might be appropriate after you both have finished a year in Pure Desire groups.)

✚ Step 1: Identify what constitutes a relapse in your mind. What type of specific behaviors create a fracture in your trust and relationship? For you, what type of behaviors are deal breakers: behaviors that would require 3-6 months of separation with the possibility of divorce?

✚ **Step 2:** Determine who your spouse needs to share their relapse with, and in what time frame. This typically includes a group member, a mentor or friend, and you. A good time frame is to share within 24 hours of the relapse.

✚ **Step 3:** Write out natural consequences of your spouse's behavior. Try to be clear about how their behavior impacts you.

✚ **Step 4:** Write out logical consequences connected to the behavior that would help you see that your spouse recognizes the serious nature of their actions. It's okay to be a bit creative and think outside the box.

Example: *a logical consequence may include forfeiting a hobby he likes (like golf) for a couple weeks. Or taking care of the kids for a day or weekend, so you can enjoy a spa day or weekend away to make self-care a priority for you.*

+ Step 5: Make a list of steps you will need to personally take in order to feel safe and stable, in preparation to fully engage in the relationship.

_____

_____

_____

_____

_____

+ Describe your desired outcome for creating this plan. If you have a clear vision of how this plan will help you rebuild trust, you are more likely to follow it. The goal of a Safety Action Plan is not punitive, but to keep you focused on what steps are needed to rebuild trust.

_____

_____

_____

_____

_____

+ What thoughts and feelings do you have about completing your Safety Action Plan?

_____

_____

_____

_____

_____

_____

✦ **Write out a prayer asking God to help you with the timing and approach to sharing your Safety Action Plan.**

You might need a pastor, counselor, or couple who has been through this process to be with you as you share it with your spouse. Part of your prayer could be asking God to prepare your husband's heart to receive it and respond well.

_____

_____

_____

_____

_____

_____

EXAMPLES OF NATURAL CONSEQUENCES WHEN A SPOUSE RELAPSES

Remember, a natural consequence occurs as a result of a choice, without anyone imposing it.

- When my spouse relapses, I feel devalued, objectified, not worth fighting for, and unprotected. I no longer feel stability in our marriage.

- When my spouse relapses, my trust is broken, and I feel vulnerable and exposed. I have a difficult time discerning what is true in our marriage and if my spouse is serious about recovery and our relationship.

- When my spouse relapses, I feel emotionally disconnected from him and no longer feel safe enough to be close and intimate.

- When my spouse lies about a relapse (including delayed confession), it creates anxiety in me that causes me to wonder what else is a lie in our marriage. I begin to replay the days and months in my head, trying to figure out what signs I missed. I start to doubt my own intuition about something being "off" in our marriage.

- When my spouse relapses, I compare myself to the person(s) my spouse fantasizes about and I feel less attractive.

- When my spouse relapses, I feel like I am not good enough.

- When my spouse relapses with porn, it is contributing to an industry that is destroying society and families.

- When my spouse relapses, it affects my relationship with God. I become distant because of the anger and isolation I feel about the situation.

- When my spouse relapses, I am not engaged with my children because my mind is preoccupied.

- When my spouse relapses, I am distracted at work and become unproductive.

- When my spouse relapses, I feel pain and insecurity.

- When my spouse is caught up in his addiction, I receive less of his energy and attention.

- When my spouse relapses, I become angry and, at times, irrational in my words and treatment of my spouse.

EXAMPLES OF LOGICAL CONSEQUENCES WHEN A RELAPSE OCCURS

These examples are tied to an action to help you understand the connection of relapse to consequences.

- Because I feel devalued and objectified after a relapse occurs, I will need space and time to process what happened. I will ask my spouse to sleep in another room, on the couch, or on the floor for _____ days/weeks until I feel safe and stable again, and ready to move forward with rebuilding trust and emotional intimacy. If relapse occurs again, the number of days out of the bed will double.

- If flirting or inappropriate behavior with a coworker takes place, I will ask my spouse not to travel alone with a coworker of the opposite sex. They will keep conversations to work topics only. If relapse continues to occur or if physical boundaries are crossed, I will ask my spouse to seek other employment or move departments.

- If my spouse misuses social media, I will ask him to delete any triggering person from his contacts and stay off social media for one month. If he keeps repeating this behavior, then I will ask him to delete his social media accounts indefinitely until he has established six months of sobriety in all areas of addiction.

- If movies are a problem, I will ask my spouse to remove his access to movies in our home. I will ask him not to rent movies alone or search any movie stories, real or online.

- If my spouse views pornography on his phone, I will ask him to block Internet access on the phone for one month. If a relapse occurs on his phone again after the month is up, I will ask him to remove Internet access until sobriety has been established for a six month period.

- If he visited a strip club, I will ask my spouse to donate $50 to an organization that rescues individuals from the sex-trafficking industry. If my spouse visits any kind of strip club or massage parlor again, the self imposed fine will double, then triple, and so on.

- If reading a sexually explicit book or magazine triggers my spouse, I will ask him to remove it from our home and only read literature that is good for personal growth.

- If my spouse crosses physical boundaries (such as kissing or other inappropriate touching), I will ask him for an immediate separation (with the possibility of divorce), and ask him to schedule a counseling appointment and call his group members. (See "If infidelity has occurred…" section.)

- Within 24 hours of disclosing the relapse, I will ask my spouse to help make arrangements for me to have time away from the kids to process and/or meet with another group member or counselor.

- After a relapse using masturbation, I will ask my spouse to sleep in a different room for two weeks. I will ask him to make an appointment with his counselor, pastor, or group leader for advice and accountability.

- I will ask my spouse to fill out a FASTER Scale weekly and share it with me.

- I will ask my spouse to seek professional counseling to help with his addiction and childhood wounds.

- I will ask my spouse to abstain from going to massage parlors of any kind.

- I will ask my spouse for access to any email or social media accounts.

- I will ask my spouse to not have any private communication (non-work-related), in any form (phone, text, instant messaging, etc.), with any person of the opposite sex, other than immediate family.

- I will ask my spouse to read healing-oriented literature about shame issues, boundaries, addiction, trauma, betrayal, and restoring trust.

- I will ask my spouse to share with our children (age-appropriate conversation) why he is not sleeping in our bedroom.

- I will ask my spouse to install pornography-blocking software on all electronic devices in our home.

- If relapse occurs on a non-essential electronic device (tablet, gaming system, etc.), I will ask my spouse to discontinue using that device for a specified period of time.

IF INFIDELITY HAS OCCURRED, I WILL ASK MY SPOUSE TO:

- Immediately schedule a counseling appointment and disclose to me and their group and/or pastor.

- Agree to not contact the other person with whom they acted out, accept any contact from them, or respond to any contact from them.

- Arrange for STD/STI testing for me and him.

- Move out of our home (or stay in another room) for a minimum of _____ months to give me time to process the affair. At the end of that time period, we will discuss the future of our marriage, which may need to be with the support of a marriage counselor. If my spouse is still involved with the individual or has not shown commitment to our marriage, I will need to seek counseling advice and initiate a separation or divorce proceedings.

- Agree to share with our children (at an age-appropriate level) why he will no longer be living in our home or bedroom.

- Agree to tell our close family, friends, and pastor what has happened, so I don't have to be the secret keeper or be the one to take on the responsibility of letting our family know what happened.

Every time a relapse occurs, the consequences should be greater than the previous time.

EXAMPLES OF STEPS YOU CAN TAKE FOR YOUR OWN PERSONAL HEALTH

- After my spouse discloses a relapse, I will immediately call _____ from my group so I can have a safe person with whom to process. This will help me avoid asking questions that are not useful for my healing, refrain from saying hurtful things that I can't take back, not shut down, and keep my mind from replaying the scenario or feeling bad about myself.

- I will pray and journal about my feelings after my spouse discloses a relapse.

- I will share with my group and tell them about the logical consequences I will implement from my Safety Action Plan in order to make sure I allow myself time to process the pain without rushing in too quickly just to "keep the peace."

- Within 24 hours of disclosing the relapse, my spouse will help arrange for me to have time away from the kids to process and/or meet with another group member.

ACTION PLAN IF SEPARATION OR DIVORCE IS NECESSARY

As you create this separation/divorce plan, incorporate any steps that are applicable from above. This plan should be used in addition to what you have already created.

✚ Create a list of items/documents you would need if leaving the house becomes necessary:

- Social Security Cards and birth certificates
- Driver's license and registration
- Insurance papers
- Medication
- Sentimental items
- School records

Action steps to secure support on the job and in public:

- Inform my boss and coworkers about my situation.
- Shop at different stores and at different hours than my spouse.

Action steps to seek support and clinical help for children to process trauma:

- Make an appointment with a family counselor.
- Ask trusted family or friends to come over to help with the kids on counseling days, court days, or other days that may be challenging for me.
- Sign up for parenting classes that deal with separation or divorce.

Create healthy boundaries regarding your spouse/ex-spouse and include consequences in your Safety Action Plan if those boundaries are crossed.

- Since relapse, my spouse and I have been living separately for 90 days while we process and rebuild trust through counseling. My spouse came inside after dropping me off at home, and we were intimate. I realize I rushed physical intimacy before regaining trust and emotional intimacy. Now I feel anxious and used again. My children are confused about us being back and forth. We will now ride separately to counseling and not be in each other's houses at night, so we can work on building trust at a healthy pace for both of us.
- I found out that my ex-spouse was out on a date. I was so hurt and angry, I shared those details and talked negatively about my ex-spouse to our children. Next time I am hurt by his actions, I will call _____ from my group to process my feelings.

- The last time I met with my ex-spouse to drop off the kids, we got into a verbal argument and called each other names in front of the kids. I will work out a plan with my ex-spouse to meet at a location of a mutual friend or family member's house until we can be around each other without reacting emotionally.

- I stay up late looking at my spouse's social media account to try to figure out what he is doing, but then I am irritable and angry with the children the next day. I will delete my social media account until I've regained stability and have processed my pain.

ACTION STEPS IF A RESTRAINING ORDER IS NEEDED

Some sexual addictions coexist with physical violence or threats. Addicts may or may not obey restraining orders. Recognize that you may need to ask the police and the court to enforce your restraining order.

I can use some or all of the following strategies to help the enforcement of my restraining order:

- Call the police if my spouse tries to contact me.

- Change the locks on my home residence.

- Keep my restraining order at _____ (safe location) and ALWAYS ON OR NEAR MY PERSON.

- I will give my restraining order to the police department in the communities I normally visit and the community where I live (including foreign countries that I travel to).

- I will inform my employer, counselor, pastor, trusted neighbor, and closest friend that I have a restraining order.

- If my spouse violates the restraining order, I can call the police and report a violation, contact my attorney, my support partner, and/or advise the court of the violation.

- If the police do not help, I can contact my attorney and file a complaint with the chief of police.

- I can also file a private criminal complaint with the district court in the jurisdiction where the violation occurred or with the district attorney. I can charge my spouse with a violation of the restraining order and all the crimes they commit in violating the order. I can call my attorney or _____ to help me with this.

- I can take a self-protection or self-defense class.

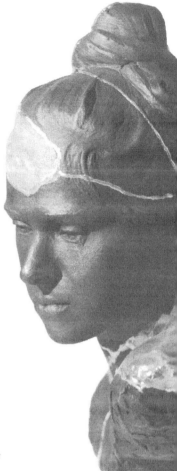

LESSON FOUR

Prioritizing Health and Wholeness

We've talked a lot about how this healing journey is a process: a series of actions or steps taken in order to achieve a specific goal. We have intentionally given you information and tools over the course of several months to help you create a strong foundation for healing. As you continue to learn more and implement specific tools into your daily lives, it will empower you to make your healing a priority.

Some tools you're already practicing include:

- **The power of gratitude:** each week writing down specific things you're thankful for and expressing this gratitude to the Lord.

- **Rehearsing of your God given promises:** when feeling the stress that often accompanies betrayal, using your personal promises from God to calm your heart and mind.

Next, we are adding **The FASTER Scale and Double Bind** exercise. These will be new tools in your toolbox that will help you become more self-aware. For a betrayed partner, when your environment becomes chaotic and feels unsafe, it may create a regression in your healing. While it would be great to think that once you start on this healing journey, you continually maintain forward motion, this is not always the case. The FASTER Scale will help you identify behaviors that are interfering with your healing and help to get you back on the path toward health and wholeness.

As long as you've known your husband, you believed certain things about him: maybe you knew he loved you, he loved the life you created together, and he would do anything to protect it. However, after discovering his hidden sexual behaviors, you are faced with a new reality. You may feel angry at being manipulated and lied to by a spouse who exploited your love for him. You may feel frustrated with how he took advantage of you and your trust in him. You might even feel resentful about all the care and compassion you put into the relationship, only to now feel used, unloved, and unappreciated.

While it has taken years to get to this place, today can be the start to living abundantly. As Jesus promised in John 10:10: *"The thief comes only to steal and kill and destroy; **I have come that they may have life, and have it to the full**."* The truth is, the future is yours: you can decide to live in the power of Christ, walk in honest relationships, and learn to love yourself as God commands.

The FASTER Scale and Double Bind

This version of The FASTER Scale has been adapted from its original form for use with betrayed partners.

The FASTER Scale,[10] created by Michael Dye, is a tool that helps us become aware of how we begin sliding into behaviors that may cause a regression in our healing. The FASTER Scale shows us how we make decisions in response to stress, which often increases isolation and minimizes how we care for ourselves.

The FASTER Scale will help us identify these behaviors and make changes, so we continue to move toward health. Moving toward health requires that we understand what it looks like to stay in restoration, and how we end up in regression, and everything in between.

 Whatever you do to speed up your body, dulls the awareness of physical and emotional pain.[11]

Each person's regression looks different. It may include aspects of excessive busyness, exercise, control, overspending, restricting food or overeating, and alcohol or drug use. It may also include self-neglect, hopelessness and depression, lashing out at the kids, or emotional affairs. There are endless pits that destroy our souls and only you thoroughly know your specific behaviors that lead to regression: behaviors and activities that pull

---

[10] Michael Dye, *The Genesis Process for Change Groups, Book Two* (Auburn: Michael Dye, 2006), 237-238.

[11] Michael Dye, Consultation, September 2022.

you away from pursuing health and wholeness. When you find yourself sliding down the slippery slope toward regression, understanding how to apply the FASTER Scale will help you stop that descent and learn how to get back to restoration.

In the following diagram, the steps leading down to regression are placed like stepping stones. As shown, the steps toward the top have more room for your feet, but those steps at the bottom can barely fit a toe, let alone give you a good grip. Imagine these stones are also wet and slippery due to the storms of life and by being blindsided by the pain and trauma of betrayal. It's easy to see how you can quickly slip into the bottom of the pit.

RESTORATION

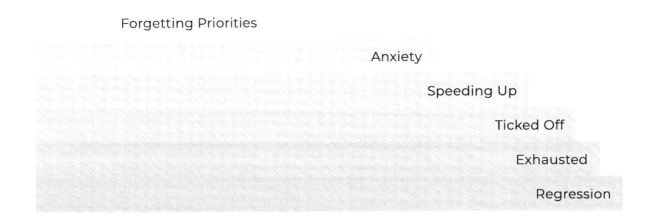

Forgetting Priorities

Anxiety

Speeding Up

Ticked Off

Exhausted

Regression

The good news is that any time you find yourself slipping down this scale, you don't have to crawl back up one step at a time. For instance, if you catch yourself feeling really angry (Ticked Off) and you want to make improvements, you don't have to move up the scale to Speeding Up, then to Anxiety, then Forgetting Priorities, until you reach Restoration. Rather, you can assess what you're feeling and why you're feeling it, which will help you to focus again on what is truly beneficial. Real breakthroughs can come when you face your feelings head on and bring them to light, so you can find solutions.

We've previously discussed how our limbic system has learned to cope with stressful situations somewhat automatically. However, as we begin healing from betrayal, we learn how to engage our prefrontal cortex and become more self-aware of what we need in the moment. The FASTER Scale will help us to recognize our stress-response behaviors and equip us to make healthy choices.

✚ When your life feels stressful, what stress-response behaviors show up?

Example: Overeating when I feel stressed and/or anxious.

_____

_____

_____

_____

_____

_____

✚ What pain and fear are you trying to avoid through this behavior?

Example: Fear of being judged or rejected if I share the pain I've experienced through betrayal.

_____

_____

_____

_____

_____

_____

_____

Because our limbic system was formed by age six, when problems came our way we didn't have an adult prefrontal cortex to problem-solve difficult situations. Our limbic brain helped us to avoid danger at all cost until the difficult situation passed. So now, as adults, this way of avoiding danger has become automatic even though, with a fully developed prefrontal cortex, we can problem-solve and come up with new solutions to best handle the situation.

To stop sliding down the FASTER Scale and process specific stressful situations, the **Double Bind** exercise will help you look at options and choose a path of action toward health rather than regression.[12] Remember, a Double Bind is where the choices available to you are difficult and will cost you something. Either choice you make will be challenging; but one will pull you further into isolation, away from relationship with God and others, and the other will push you toward relationship with God and others. Even if the choices are both difficult, the direction they take you is key to your healing. The Double Bind helps you face the fear of doing the hard thing to resolve the stressful situation.

Starting next week you will have a new FASTER Scale in your *Journal*. The purpose is to monitor where you are on a weekly basis and do a Double Bind exercise to help you get back to Restoration.

For this week, we will walk through each step and identify the behaviors or attitudes that are typical in each category. Each person's experience is different; so as we go step by step, you will be asked to circle the behaviors or attitudes you have experienced in the last week.

Note: Some personal commentary has been added to better describe each category. You can circle some of those comments as well as what is listed for each of the FASTER acrostic letters.

FASTER SCALE

Created by Michael Dye from *The Genesis Process*.

Adapted by Pure Desire Ministries with permission from Michael Dye, *The Genesis Process*.

R estoration – **(Accepting life on God's terms, with trust, grace, mercy, vulnerability and gratitude.)** No current secrets; working to resolve problems; identifying fears and feelings; keeping commitments to meetings, prayer, family, church, people, goals, and self; being open and honest, making eye contact; increasing in relationships with God and others; true accountability.

✚ **Circle each behavior in Restoration that you experienced in the last week.**

This is where we want to live. When we live in Restoration, it allows us to live our lives trusting God and trusting those people closest to us. However, living in Restoration becomes threatened by our circumstances, impacted by external situations and how we internally process the pain and trauma of that situation. When we experience the devastation of betrayal, the stress, pain, and trauma can cause us to begin sliding down The FASTER Scale.

---

[12] Dye, *The Genesis Process*, 45.

✛ List two or three actions that help you stay in Restoration.

01. _____

02. _____

03. _____

F orgetting Priorities – (Feeling powerless to change the present circumstances and moving away from trusting God. Denial, flight, a change in what's important; how you spend your time, energy, and thoughts.) Secrets; less time/energy for God, meetings, church; avoiding group support; superficial conversations; sarcasm; isolating; changes in goals; obsessed with relationships; breaking promises and commitments; neglecting family; lack of self-care; preoccupation with material things, TV, computers, entertainment; procrastination; lying; overconfidence.

Example: *I don't take time to do the things I know are important. Since I've experienced betrayal, there has been a shift in my priorities. I begin to run away from my personal problems, focusing more on other people (including the addict) and other things.*

✛ Under Forgetting Priorities, circle the behaviors you experienced in the last week.

✛ What does Forgetting Priorities usually look like for you?

_____

_____

_____

_____

_____

_____

_____

_____

_____

_____

Forgetting Priorities will lead to the inclusion of:

A nxiety – **(Consumed by negative thoughts and undefined fear; getting energy from emotions.)** Worry, using profanity, being fearful; being resentful; replaying old, negative thoughts; perfectionism; judging other's motives; making goals and lists that you can't complete; mind reading; fantasy; hypervigilance; sleep problems; trouble concentrating; seeking/creating drama; gossip; using over-the-counter medication for pain, sleep or weight control; suspiciousness; catastrophic thinking.

Example: *I'm preoccupied with my husband's behavior, which causes me to excessively worry and creates anxiety. All my energy is put into making sure he doesn't mess up so I don't get hurt again.*

✚ Under Anxiety, circle the behaviors you experienced in the last week.

✚ What does Anxiety usually look like for you ?

_____

_____

_____

_____

_____

_____

Anxiety then leads to the inclusion of:

S peeding Up – **(Trying to outrun the anxiety which is usually the first sign of depression.)** Super busy and always in a hurry (finding good reason to justify the work); workaholic; can't relax; avoiding slowing down; feeling driven; can't turn off thoughts; skipping meals; binge eating (usually at night); experiencing false guilt; overspending; can't identify own feelings/needs; repetitive negative thoughts; irritable; dramatic mood swings; too much caffeine; over exercising; nervousness; difficulty being alone and/or with people; difficulty listening to others; avoiding support; making excuses for having to "do it all."

Example: *I'm overwhelmed with trying to navigate life after betrayal. If I can stay busy, I won't have time to think about what's happening to my world. And then I won't have to feel the effects of my world crumbling.*

✚ Under Speeding Up, circle the behaviors you experienced in the last week.

✚ What does Speeding Up usually look like for you?

_____

_____

_____

_____

_____

Speeding Up then leads to the inclusion of:

Ticked Off – (Getting adrenaline high on anger and aggression.) Procrastination causing crisis in money, work, and relationships; increased sarcasm; black and white (all or nothing) thinking; feeling alone; nobody understands; overreacting; road rage; constant resentments; pushing others away; increasing isolation; blaming; arguing; irrational thinking; can't take criticism; defensive; people avoiding you; needing to be right; digestive problems; headaches; obsessive (stuck) thoughts; can't forgive; feeling superior; using intimidation; seeking confrontation; passive-aggressive behaviors; thoughts of getting even/revenge.

Example: *I'm so angry! I gave him the best years of my life and he cheated on me. Although he confessed and is in a recovery group, I don't buy it. He's probably lying and manipulating them too.*

✚ Under Ticked Off, circle the behaviors you experienced in the last week.

✚ What does Ticked Off usually look like for you?

_____

_____

_____

_____

_____

Ticked Off then leads to the inclusion of:

E xhausted – **(Loss of physical and emotional energy; coming off the adrenaline high, and the onset of depression.)** Depressed; panicked; confused; hopelessness; sleeping too much or too little; can't cope; overwhelmed; crying for "no reason"; can't think; forgetful; pessimistic; helpless; tired; numb; wanting to run; constant cravings for old coping behaviors; thinking of using sex, drugs, or alcohol; really isolating; people angry with you; self abuse; suicidal thoughts; spontaneous crying; no goals; survival mode; not returning phone calls; missing work; irritability; no appetite; feeling powerless; victim mentality; short-term memory loss.

Example: *I can no longer keep up with the busyness. I feel hopeless, depressed, overwhelmed, and extremely sad. My mind is consumed with dark thinking. I've kept myself totally isolated from others and continue to think, "What's the use?" I wish there was a way to escape or run away from the pain.*

✚ **Under Exhausted, circle the behaviors you experienced in the last week.**

✚ **What does Exhausted usually look like for you ?**

_____

_____

_____

_____

_____

Exhausted then leads to the inclusion of:

R egression – **(Stalled or moving backward in your healing.)** Feeling unsafe; unable to regulate emotions; sleep disturbances (sleeping too much or too little); ruminating about discovery/disclosure; feeling unusually fearful; binge eating; using alcohol and drugs to cope; symptoms of physical distress: headaches, stomach aches, nausea; easily startled; anorexia; bulimia; flirting; obsessed with social media; unable to trust God and others. For divorced partners: engaging in new relationships without support/accountability.

Regression may feel like your healing progress has stalled, is moving backward, or spinning in circles with no forward motion. The pain and trauma of betrayal is consuming your mind, body, and soul.

✚ Under Regression, circle the behaviors you experienced in the last week.

✚ What does Regression usually look like for you?

_____

_____

_____

_____

_____

_____

_____

_____

_____

_____

_____

_____

_____

_____

_____

_____

_____

As stated before, a Double Bind is a lose/lose situation: when the choices available to you are equally difficult. The situation will not be resolved on its own, but will become more intense if left unaddressed. This will often make your internal conflict greater. At this point, you usually slide quickly down the FASTER Scale toward regression. However, facing your fear and doing the hard thing is the best choice for finding a resolution and continuing on your journey toward health.

Look at the following examples for a better understanding of how to use the Double Bind exercise.

DOUBLE BIND EXAMPLES

Choices	Apply Formula		Plan	
Problem/ Situation	**If I do... (face the problem)**	**If I don't... (avoid the problem)**	**The right thing is the hard thing to do**	**What, when, who, where, and how ?**
Seems like my spouse is more isolated, procrastinating on chores, and putting off promises to the kids. Concerned he has relapsed.	*I need to face my fear of confrontation and talk to him about his behaviors, and be prepared to follow through with consequences if he has relapsed.*	*I will continue to feel anxious and wonder if he's relapsed. I will regress in my own healing. He may relapse, requiring the need to have consequences anyway.*	*Face my fear, consider what consequences I need to enforce and other possible outcomes if he's relapsed. I need to identify specific issues and choose a time to discuss it with him.*	*Journal my concerns within two days and get support from friends. Schedule a meeting with him alone and away from our homes within three days.*
I feel panicked and stressed about my husband's work trip. He often acted out when away from home. I'm so worried it will happen again.	*I need to talk with him about my concerns before his trip. If he relapses, I will need to follow through with my Safety Action Plan.*	*I will experience more physical symptoms of anxiety and stress. I will be consumed with his possible relapse and become irritable with the kids.*	*Journal about my feelings, fears. Discuss with safe friends for input. Be intentional about making time to talk before his trip.*	*Journal, pray about it, and reach out for support from friends. Make time to talk with him several days before his trip, so we can be in a healthy place before he leaves.*

Choices	Apply Formula		Plan	
Problem/ Situation	If I do... (face the problem)	If I don't... (avoid the problem)	The right thing is the hard thing to do	What, when, who, where, and how?
I found porn on his phone. When I confronted him, he lied about it. He later confessed that he's been struggling for the past year.	If our marriage is going to last, we need something more, that will get to the core of his issues. We need counseling. I don't know how we'll afford it or make time for it.	Our marriage won't last. Without a major change, I'm filing for divorce. I can't keep doing this... each time the pain is worse than the time before. It's killing me.	I will share this with my group for prayer/ support. I will research specific counseling programs that deal with porn issues. I will talk with my husband about our options and a plan to move forward.	I'll share this with my group today. This week, I will do research and make a list of potential counseling options. I will schedule time next week to talk with my husband about the options and determine a plan.

✚ Of the Double Bind examples given, which situation listed resonates with you most? Explain.

_____

_____

_____

_____

Note: If you are feeling triggered by any of the lesson content or this healing process, and want to pursue professional help, please contact Pure Desire at 503-489-0230 or visit **puredesire.org/counseling**.

5

CHAPTER FIVE

Why Does
He Do This ?

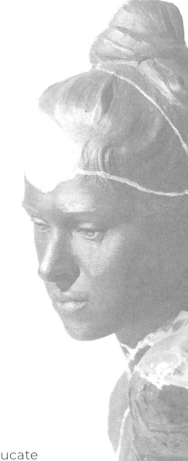

Understanding Addiction and Recovery

As a woman who has experienced betrayal, it is important for you to educate yourself about compulsive sexual behaviors and the impact this has had on your husband. The information presented in the lessons in this chapter are to help you understand the foundational pieces that contribute to sex addiction. Chances are your husband has been in those murky waters of bondage for years and he needs to pull anchor and move into the clear waters of truth. By understanding his recovery process, it will help you assess where he's at and determine if he is getting better.

This is not intended to minimize, justify, or excuse his behavior. This is for you. So you have accurate information about the nature of compulsive sexual behaviors and can make informed decisions about your future.

What is Sex Addiction/ Compulsive Sexual Behavior?

According to a definition commonly used in clinical settings, sex addiction (as well as compulsive sexual behaviors) can be described as "...an unhealthy relationship to any sexual experience (thoughts, fantasies, activities, etc.) that a person continues to engage in despite adverse consequences."[1]

---

[1] Stefanie Carnes, *Mending a Shattered Heart: A Guide for Partners of Sex Addicts* (Carefree: Gentle Path Press, 2011), 9.

The following ten criteria are key to diagnosing sex addiction.[2] If someone meets three or more of these criteria, and has struggled for six months or more, they would be considered a sex addict. This diagnosis should be obtained through an experienced, trained professional clinician, who is equipped to evaluate and determine whether or not a person is a sex addict.

01. Recurrent failure to resist sexual impulses in order to engage in specific sexual behaviors

02. Frequently engaging in those behaviors to a greater extent or over a longer period of time than intended

03. Persistent desire or unsuccessful efforts to stop, reduce, or control these behaviors

04. Inordinate amounts of time spent in obtaining sex, being sexual, or recovering from sexual experiences

05. Preoccupation with sexual behavior or preparatory activities

06. Frequently engaging in the behavior when expected to fulfill occupational, academic, domestic, or social obligations

07. Continuation of the behavior despite knowledge of having a persistent or recurrent social, financial, psychological, or physical problem that is caused or exacerbated by the behavior

08. The need to increase the intensity, frequency, number, or risk level of behaviors in order to achieve the desired effect; or diminished effect with continued behaviors at the same level of intensity, frequency, number, or risk

09. Giving up or limiting social, occupational, or recreational activities because of the behavior

10. Distress, anxiety, restlessness, or irritability if unable to engage in the behavior

The purpose of sharing this information is so that you will have a full understanding of sex addiction. As you can see, there is a progressive nature to this addiction. To some extent, especially early on, most addict's think they can control their behavior. What they quickly learn is that it begins to take over and control their behaviors, creating a compulsive pattern of acting out, increased shame, and deep despair.

Rarely, does anyone set out to become a sex addict. At some point, perhaps as a young boy, your husband found a stash of his father's pornography hidden in the garage. Or when rummaging through the town's dump with his friends, found pornographic magazines that had been thrown away. Or, had a sexual encounter with a neighbor friend, which left him curious and confused. Or maybe he experienced some form of sexual abuse, which created excruciating pain and trauma that no young boy should ever experience. Possibly he was neglected or mistreated. Perhaps

---

[2] Carnes, *Mending a Shattered Heart*, 10.

he was physically punished and abused for things he didn't do and can't make sense of it to this day. Maybe a parent died or his parents divorced, which left him feeling abandoned and alone.

It is these types of life experiences, and countless others, that contribute to sex addiction. Dr. Patrick Carnes, a leading expert on sex addiction, suggests that fear of abandonment and shame play a significant role in a sex addict's life.

Addicts, at one level, judge themselves by society's standards. Unable to measure up to these, they live with constant pain and alienation. Each one, convinced that he or she alone is afflicted, lives in isolation and constant fear of discovery. Addicts withhold a major portion of themselves–a pain deeply felt, but never expressed or witnessed. They do not trust nor do they become intimate with others, especially their families. There is the possibility that family members will find out about their behaviors and the certainty that if that happens they would leave the addict. As we shall see, fear of abandonment and shame are at the core of addiction. The alienation becomes a quagmire within which addicts struggle, only to become more isolated.[3]

At some point in your husband's life, something happened to him or around him that felt out of control. It could have been one major event or several events that happened over a period of time which left him feeling hurt, broken, alone, afraid, responsible, and more. And because no one wants to feel these things, especially if we can't make sense of them, our normal response is to want to do something to make ourselves feel better. To take away or escape the painful things we're feeling. Something that will medicate and relieve our pain, even if it's just for a moment. This is what sex addiction is about.

Note: *While the above described experiences would be awful for anyone, it does not excuse your husband's behaviors and the impact his choices have had on you.* **This is not to excuse the behavior, but to explain the behavior. Having this explanation will help you make informed decisions about your future.**

Just as we learned the Stages of Healing for those who have experienced betrayal, there are Stages of Recovery for those who struggle with sex addiction/compulsive sexual behaviors.

Stages of Recovery

When considering the Stages of Recovery, here are two things to keep in mind:
1) The addict needs to be more committed to recovery than to his addiction;
2) True transforming change takes three to five years.[4]

---

[3] Patrick Carnes, *Out of the Shadows: Understanding Sexual Addiction* (Center City: Hazelden, 2001), 6.

[4] Patrick Carnes, *Don't Call It Love: Recovery From Sexual Addiction* (New York: Bantam Books, 1991), 236.

Recovery happens in stages:[5]

- Break denial and admit the person really does need help to change
- Understand The Cyclone of Addiction and how the brain has been hijacked
- Surrender to a process of change and commitment to sobriety
- Access the wounds that drive the addiction
- Grieve the loss
- Repair damaged relationships and rebuild intimacy
- Maintain a healthy lifestyle

STAGE ONE: BREAKING DENIAL

Strong walls of denial can take months to break. Denial has allowed the addict to be subjective when it comes to evaluating his actions. He has had to rationalize his actions over the years and has ignored any objective standard that would help him see clearly. In some cases, especially if the addict has put his wife at risk for HIV or other sexually transmitted diseases, a polygraph test can give the wife a bottom line. The test helps the wife know the extent of the addiction and gives the addict an objective tool to evaluate his actions. (See the appendix, page 326 for more information on the polygraph test.) Scripture declares the truth will set you free (John 8:31-32) and this powerfully applies to the addict's life. **Until all secrets are exposed, he cannot experience full freedom.**

✛ Based on your situation, circle the percentage of the betrayal that you think has been revealed.

10%   25%   50%   75%   100%

✛ What do you think it will take for more truth to be disclosed?

---

[5] These stages represent the seven pillars men walk through in the *Seven Pillars of Freedom Workbook.*

STAGE TWO: UNDERSTANDING THE CYCLONE OF ADDICTION AND HOW THE BRAIN HAS BEEN HIJACKED

The addict realizes the nature of his addiction and why his strategy of trying harder on his own over the years has not and will not work. (Romans 7:15 – I do what I don't want to do and don't do what I want to do.)

STAGE THREE: SURRENDERING TO A PROCESS OF CHANGE AND COMMITMENT TO SOBRIETY

The addict's commitment to a Pure Desire recovery group breaks isolation and his commitment to renew his mind will bring change (Romans 12:2). This commitment takes time and effort. It will take consistent, daily recovery work for his mind to be renewed.

STAGE FOUR: ACCESSING THE WOUNDS THAT DRIVE THE ADDICTION

Early childhood or adolescent trauma and/or abuse often contributes to the creation of addictive coping behaviors to survive. At Pure Desire, we have found that at least 80% of male addicts have a deep father wound. As a result of deep wounds, most men feel worthless or unloved. Part of healing those deep wounds is getting in touch with the lies that are attached to the wounds and replacing those lies with the truth of who God says he is.

STAGE FIVE: GRIEVING THE LOSS

This may include grieving the loss of having a healthy, supportive family growing up. Or grieving the loss of innocence as abuse is acknowledged. Statistics show that the majority of sexual addicts have been emotionally (97%), physically (72%), and/or sexually (81%) abused.[6]

STAGE SIX: REPAIRING DAMAGED RELATIONSHIPS AND BUILDING INTIMACY

Addicts usually have an attachment and intimacy disorder. In other words, they have never learned how to be in a healthy relationship. Through his group experience, he will begin to learn empathy as he shares and hears other's stories. He will be challenged to repair relationships and learn to pursue his wife. He may also need to repair relationships with his children and other relatives.

---

[6] Carnes, *Don't Call It Love*, 146.

STAGE SEVEN: MAINTAINING A HEALTHY LIFESTYLE

This will require the addict to continue in the healing process a minimum of three to five years. The *Seven Pillars of Freedom Workbook* is designed to help men move through these phases and work toward a healthy lifestyle. Men are encouraged not only to go through a group, but also co-lead a group the next year and lead a group the following year. When addicts "pay it forward" and commit to a group long term, they break isolation and develop empathy and healthy attachment. When sobriety is established, they need to be held accountable for doing things that will reflect healthy behaviors, which will allow them to connect more deeply with their wife and children.

✛ If your spouse has started his recovery journey, what stage best describes where he is at this point in time? Explain.

_____

_____

_____

_____

Why three to five years?

Recovery not only happens in stages, but also in layers, much like peeling layers of an onion. Both you and your spouse may feel like you are moving backward at times, but in reality, sometimes you have to recycle back through some of the stages to pick up the loose ends, as demonstrated by the following diagram:

THE RECOVERY PROCESS[7]

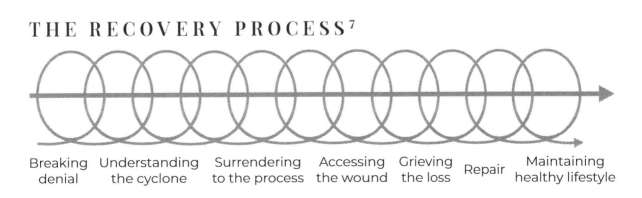

| Breaking denial | Understanding the cyclone | Surrendering to the process | Accessing the wound | Grieving the loss | Repair | Maintaining healthy lifestyle |

---

[7] Ted Roberts, *Hope For Men* (Gresham, Oregon: East Hill Church, 1993), 10.

A word of advice for you and your husband: be patient with the process. On this healing and recovery journey, new issues may surface and make it seem as though you are regressing. The truth is that you are dealing with deep issues and **there is no quick fix**.

Many people have traumatic experiences in life that result in unwanted behaviors; the things we chose to do, at the time, to medicate our pain. Some people choose drugs and/or alcohol to medicate their pain. Some people choose food to medicate their pain: either overeating or starving themselves when life feels out of control. Some people look to video games, gambling, shopping...whatever it takes, in the moment, to make themselves feel better. To escape the feeling, the reminder of our past pain and trauma, that has surfaced once again.

✚ Are you aware of any significant traumatic event(s) that happened in your husband's life? Explain.

_____

_____

_____

_____

_____

_____

_____

_____

This does not, in any way, minimize, justify, or excuse your husband's behaviors. Not at all. There is no excuse for what he has done. There is no justification for the pain and trauma you're feeling right now. And providing this information and a greater understanding of compulsive sexual behaviors will not minimize the impact his choices and behaviors have had on you.

The primary purpose of this information is to help you make informed decisions about your life and future. Another reason is to help you recognize your need for grace in this process. Grace for yourself (and eventually grace for your husband).

So let us come boldly to the throne of our gracious God. There we will receive his mercy, and we will find grace to help us when we need it most.

HEBREWS 4:16 (NLT)

It is imperative that we understand our need for grace in this healing process.

✚ How have you seen God's grace at work in your healing process? Explain.

_____

_____

_____

_____

_____

_____

_____

_____

_____

_____

✚ In what ways does this Scripture give you comfort and hope for your healing?

_____

_____

_____

_____

_____

_____

_____

_____

_____

_____

_____

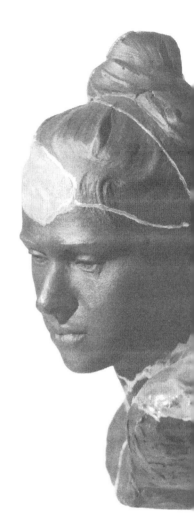

LESSON TWO

How Sexual Addiction Affects the Brain

People often ask, "Is sexual addiction a disorder or a sin?" The answer: YES. The following explanation of the spiritual battle and the neurochemistry of the brain will help you better understand why sexual addiction is such a struggle.[8]

As a Christian, we know that the experiences we have on this earth have a spiritual component to them. Some would describe this as a spiritual war or battle.

The New Testament only uses the term "war" or "warfare" five times, but its focus is intriguing. Let's quickly look at each incident so you have a clear understanding of the spiritual battle that surrounds all Christians.

> *For though we live in the world, we do not wage war as the world does. The weapons we fight with are not the weapons of the world. On the contrary, they have divine power to demolish strongholds. We demolish arguments and every pretension that sets itself up against the knowledge of God, and we take captive every thought to make it obedient to Christ.*
>
> 2 CORINTHIANS 10:3-5 (NIV)

---

[8] Ted Roberts, *Seven Pillars of Freedom Workbook* (Gresham: Pure Desire Ministries International, 2009), 23-28.

This is Paul's classic statement about the nature of the spiritual battle every Christ-follower faces. This war he speaks of is about pulling down strongholds of the mind. The focus is not on Satan, but rather on taking charge of our minds and taking our thoughts captive for the glory of God.

> *Timothy, my son, I am giving you this command in keeping with the prophecies once made about you, so that by recalling them you may fight the battle well,*
>
> 1 TIMOTHY 1:18 (NIV)

Paul is challenging his apprentice to stay in the fight and to be faithful to his calling. Once again the focus is not on the devil, but on Timothy's mind.

> *No one serving as a soldier gets entangled in civilian affairs, but rather tries to please his commanding officer.*
>
> 2 TIMOTHY 2:4 (NIV)

Paul is calling Timothy to clear out the clutter in his life and to be single-minded. He is exhorting him to stay committed to the call of God regardless of the cost, and to focus his mind.

> *What causes fights and quarrels among you? Don't they come from your desires that battle within you?*
>
> JAMES 4:1 (NIV)

James is calling the reader to not be controlled by the self-oriented thinking that can so easily become part of our daily thought process.

> *Dear friends, I urge you, as foreigners and exiles, to abstain from sinful desires, which wage war against your soul.*
>
> 1 PETER 2:11 (NIV)

Once again, the focus is on dealing with a self-orientated way of thinking that can tear apart a person's soul.

This is crucial to grasp because **sexual addiction is all about self-focus and everything revolving around the addict.**

As a betrayed partner, this is not new information. Even if you didn't know how to explain your husband's behaviors, or know why he behaved the way he did, you have lived with a person who was self-focused and everything revolved around him.

Again, the purpose of giving you this information is not to excuse your husband's behaviors or minimize how you've been hurt through betrayal. **This is for you.** It is intended to give you a greater understanding of how the human brain works and how it is affected by sexually addictive behaviors.

The previous Scriptures describe a spiritual battle or war that affects our mind and our way of thinking. Therefore, if the battlefield is in our mind, especially for those struggling with compulsive sexual behaviors, it becomes even more important to understand brain function and how it's impacted by addiction.

The Brain

The human brain is one of God's most mysterious creations. It contains approximately 100 billion nerve cells or what is commonly referred to as **neurons**.[9] A single neuron communicates or sends information by passing a chemical—**a neurotransmitter**—to another neuron. The connections between neurons—**the synapse or synaptic gap**—can span from 10 trillion to 100 trillion points of contact within the human nervous system.

Neurons

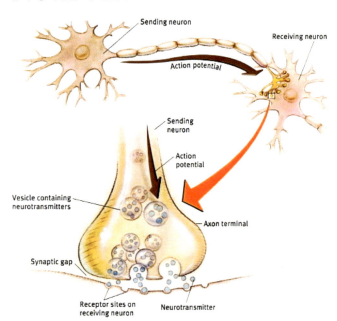

[10]The primary function of a neuron is to process information.[11] Neurons vary in both form and size depending on their specific function; some less than fractions of an inch and others up to three feet in length. **They are also specific to which type of neurotransmitter they respond: dopamine, serotonin, or norepinephrine, for example.**

---

[9] Jackson Beatty, *The Human Brain: Essentials of Behavioral Neuroscience* (Thousand Oaks: Sage Publications, Inc., 2001), 1.

[10] Hall, R. AP Psychology course. http://www.rhsmpsychology.com/Handouts/synapse.htm

[11] Beatty, *The Human Brain*, 31.

Brain Synapse

Here's what is happening in a healthy brain. In very simple terms, an electrical impulse travels down the **axon**, producing a chemical reaction—releasing neurotransmitters into the synaptic gap. A receptor on the receiving cell will bind to a specific neurotransmitter, in many ways reflecting a lock-and-key scenario, absorbing the neurotransmitter, yielding a specific action. This is called **synaptic transmission**. The excess neurotransmitters not used by the receiving cell are taken back into the sending cell—recycled—through a reuptake process for repackaging and reuse.[12] Although this process is extremely complex, down to the most minuscule detail, it is important to understand how these mechanisms work in connection to addictive behavior.

✚ In your own words, write out the key function of these terms to help you remember their significance.

Neurons: _____

Neurotransmitters: _____

Synapse/Synaptic Gap: _____

The Limbic System

The limbic system includes a collection of structures associated with processing emotion, mood, and memory.[13] Three specific areas of the brain play a significant role in addictive behavior.

We've previously discussed these areas of the brain (Chapter 2, Lesson 2), but let's review:

- The **prefrontal cortex** receives information from the limbic system and

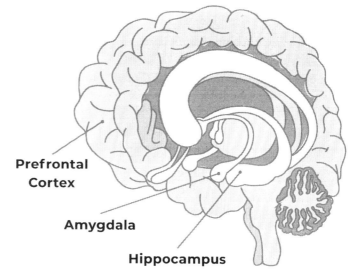

Prefrontal Cortex

Amygdala

Hippocampus

---

[12] Beatty, *The Human Brain*, 115.

[13] Peter Abrahams, *How the Brain Works: Understanding Brain Function, Thought, and Personality*. (New York: Metro Books, 2015), 28-29.

other parts of the brain. When it comes to addictive behaviors, it is instrumental in decision making, planning, problem solving, and impulse control.

- The **amygdala** is involved in emotional processing and regulation, especially critical to our fear response.
- The **hippocampus** is all about memory formation, retention, and recall.

When we have an experience, especially an event that is perceived as threatening or dangerous, the hippocampus and the amygdala work together to process the event—the specific details of what happened and the way it made us feel are stored together in our limbic system.

The disconnect: research suggests that the limbic system—the emotional center of the brain—is fully functional by age six.[14] However, the prefrontal cortex—decision-making, planning, and impulse control—is not fully developed until the mid-twenties.

The reality of this physiological disconnect: most of us will spend almost 20 years interpreting our world—what is happening to us and around us—through a highly emotional filter; through a limbic filter. Not because we are overreacting or overly emotional, but because our brain is not yet capable of rational thought.

✚ **In your own words, briefly describe the function of these areas of the brain.**

Prefrontal cortex: _____

Hippocampus: _____

Amygdala: _____

God designed our limbic system for survival, to help us develop awareness and learn from our environment—whether we are safe or in danger. Collectively, the areas of the limbic system work together to influence and create emotion, mood, and memory. In response to an emotional trigger—a limbic reaction, if you will—the limbic system will set in motion a sequence of neurological actions.

If a situation is alarming or frightening, it will trigger our fight-flight-or-freeze response.[15] If we encounter a person as a friend, our memory will override the need or feeling to retreat, and produce the appropriate warm-hearted response.

---

[14] BetterHelp, *Adolescent Brain Development And What It Means*, 2018. https://www.betterhelp.com/advice/adolescence/adolescent-brain-development-and-what-it-means/.

[15] Daniel J. Siegel, *Pocket Guide to Interpersonal Neurobiology: An Integrative Handbook of the Mind* (New York: W.W. Norton & Company, Inc., 2012), 12-1.

When it comes to understanding how the limbic system works, you may know exactly what this feels like. The day you discovered your husband's secret life and his struggle with hidden sexual behaviors are captured in this area of your brain. The hippocampus gathered specific details about the event—where you were, who else was there, what you were wearing, the weather outside—and the amygdala captured how you felt in the moment—pain, heartache, devastated, humiliated, shocked—and now these things are stored together in your brain.

Later, if something triggers a memory of this event, we will experience the same feelings we did when the event originally happened, even if we don't recognize it. For example, for a betrayed partner, a basketball game can be a trigger or provoke an emotional response if that is where she learned of her husband's affair.

Our limbic system is so important. If it is the filter by which we process everything that's happening to us and around us, especially during our younger years when our prefrontal cortex is not fully developed, what happens when we experience trauma? What if we have been physically, emotionally, or sexually abused? As mentioned before, Dr. Patrick Carnes' research found a common theme of abuse among thousands who struggled with sexual addiction: 81% had been sexually abused, 72% had been physically abused, and 97% had been emotionally abused.

Many people who struggle with compulsive sexual behaviors have experienced trauma in the form of neglect, poverty, bullying, racism, or feeling marginalized. They may have been raised in an environment where they didn't feel safe talking to their parents about what was happening to them. So they internalized their pain and looked for ways to medicate their feelings in order to survive.

We have learned that trauma is not just an event that took place sometime in the past; it is also the imprint left by that experience on mind, brain, and body. This imprint has ongoing consequences for how the human organism manages to survive in the present.[16]

✚ **To your knowledge, has your husband experienced any of these forms of trauma ?**

_____

_____

_____

_____

[16] Bessel van der Kolk, *The Body Keeps the Score: Brain, Mind, and Body in the Healing of Trauma* (New York: Penguin Books, 2014), 21.

This is why understanding how the limbic system works is so important. For many people who struggle with addictive behaviors, the things they experienced in their younger years left an imprint on their mind, brain, and body. Even the things that happened beyond their control left a mark: the sudden death of a parent or family member; having to move schools; divorce; quitting college to support your siblings; not receiving attention from parents. Whatever it was, disrupted their ability to process their world in a healthy way. Which, for many, left them searching for a way to medicate their hidden pain.

This is why we often say, **"Sexual addiction is not about sex. It's about medicating pain."**

Somewhere in your husband's past, he experienced some form of pain and trauma that left brokenness. Never learning to manage stress and pain in a healthy way has led him to cope and escape in ways that are harmful to himself and the people around him. This, in no way, excuses, minimizes, or justifies his behavior. However, it might help to explain his behavior.

✚ Can you think of one or two painful and/or traumatic events your husband experienced that could be currently affecting him?

✚ What negative patterns have you observed in your husband's attempt to medicate the pain of these experiences?

✚ What did you learn about the brain and how it's impacted by sexual addiction?

✚ What does having this information do for you and your healing journey?

✚ If you feel ready, write a prayer for your spouse, possibly using some of the Scriptures at the beginning of this lesson. You can't change him, but you can advocate on his behalf.

_____

_____

_____

_____

_____

_____

_____

_____

_____

_____

✚ If you are separated or divorced, how can you contend for the addict in light of what your children need in a godly dad?

_____

_____

_____

_____

_____

_____

_____

_____

_____

✝ Write a prayer for yourself, asking God to increase your awareness of what's happening to you spiritually, emotionally, and mentally; and for protection over your mind, body, and soul. You too are in a battle where the enemy is using the trauma of betrayal against you.

How a Sex Addict's Brain is Hijacked

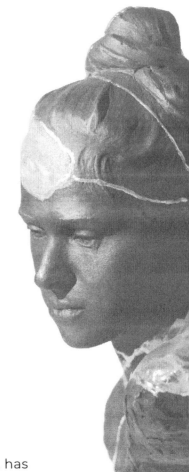

The brain can be reclaimed and renewed to a place of health, even if it has been hijacked by addictive behavior.[17] Understanding how the limbic system works in connection to addiction and compulsive sexual behaviors has been influential in helping many partners recognize that their husband's behaviors are not the result of anything they did or didn't do. While it doesn't excuse, minimize, or justify any of their husband's behaviors, having this information often helps facilitate healing for partners.

In the last lesson, we discussed the limbic system and the role it plays in capturing significant events, how we feel in the moment, and storing these things together in our brain (the amygdala and hippocampus specifically).

In this lesson, we're going to dig deeper into what's happening in the brain and limbic system when it comes to addictive behaviors.

---

[17] John Ratey, *A User's Guide to the Brain: Perception, Attention, and the Four Theaters of the Brain* (New York: Vintage Books, 2001), 227.

The Reward System[18]

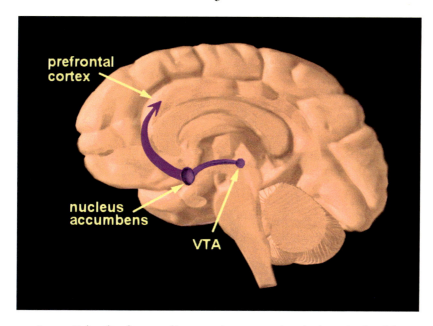

Everything we do—all of our thoughts, feelings, and behaviors—originate in our brain. The motivation behind *why we do what we do* happens through a specific process. Here's how this works.

The ventral tegmental area (VTA) is highly responsive to the production of dopamine.[19] This is the origin of the dopamine system. It looks for excitement or novelty (stimulation) in our environment. Once it finds excitement, the release of dopamine increases and is projected to various regions of the brain: **the nucleus accumbens, amygdala, and hippocampus of the limbic system, and the prefrontal cortex.**

When dopamine is stimulated in the brain, it creates feelings of euphoria and pleasure. Who doesn't want that! When we participate in behaviors that stimulate the production of dopamine in our brain, we naturally want to repeat those behaviors. The reward system doesn't just create feelings of pleasure. It includes areas of the brain involved with motivation and memory. Logically, we determine that if we continue the same behaviors, we will get the same response. If it were only that simple.

Dopamine is a powerful motivator. In laboratory studies, rats will perform a specific action to receive an electrical stimulation to their brain—rewarding them with the production of dopamine—ignoring all other rewards such as food and water.[20] When it comes to stimulating the production of dopamine, rats will press a lever as rapidly as 2,000 times per hour, each time receiving an electrical stimulation. In fact, they will continue to press the lever at this same rate for 24 hours or more. This is just one example of the power of dopamine.

---

[18] Reward Pathway. http://www.drugabuse.gov/pubs/teaching/Teaching2.html

[19] Jackson Beatty, *Principles of Behavioral Neuroscience* (Dubuque: Wm. C. Brown Communications, Inc., 1995), 348.

[20] Beatty, *Principles of Behavioral Neuroscience*, 346-347.

This also helps to explain why stopping compulsive sexual behaviors is so challenging. The person who struggles has created a condition by which their brain has developed more of an automatic response to the threat of pain. It becomes sort of an "A + B = C" scenario. "If I feel stressed at work (A), and look at porn and masturbate (B), then I will feel momentary relief from my pain (C)."

✚ **When have you observed this type of "A + B = C" scenario play out in your husband's behaviors? Briefly explain the situation (which may or may not be related to his sexually addictive behaviors).**

_____

_____

_____

_____

When you are struggling with sexual bondage, your prefrontal cortex commitment to Christ is usually being pulled off course by the autopilot of your limbic system deep within your brain. When you continue to make choices that don't make any sense in your life, when you repeatedly make destructive sexual decisions, then mark it down. **It is a limbic system problem.**[21]

This quote speaks to the disconnect between the prefrontal cortex, the rational part of the brain, and the limbic system, which is an emotional part of the brain. It's a perfect reminder that sexual brokenness has more to do with medicating the emotional pain and wounds people have experienced, than it has to do with sex.

While compulsive sexual behaviors have a clear physiological impact, there is also a spiritual component that cannot be ignored.

> For the desires of the flesh are against the Spirit, and the desires of the Spirit are against the flesh, for these are opposed to each other, to keep you from doing the things you want to do.
>
> GALATIANS 5:17 (ESV)

The process of recovery and renewing the mind is both spiritual and physical. It's about recognizing how sex addiction has created chaos in the brain of an addict and inviting the Holy Spirit to speak life and truth into these broken areas of their life.

---

[21] Ted Roberts, *Seven Pillars of Freedom* (Gresham: Pure Desire Ministries International, 2009), 232.

✚ How has learning about the limbic system given you more understanding of and/or insight into your husband's behaviors? Explain.

The Addicted Brain[22]

Have you ever thought of addictive behavior as learned behavior? Think about this: learning produces changes in the way we think, feel, and act.[23] When our behavior is reinforced with a positive result—making us feel in control, happy, or safe—we naturally want to repeat the behaviors that created this specific response. The more we repeat the behavior, the more it changes our brain, strengthening neural connections.

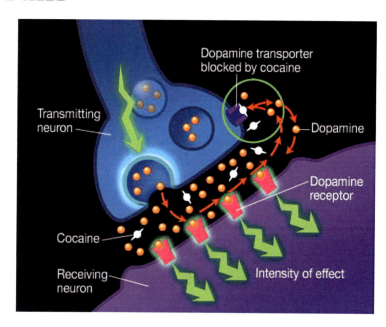

In the previous lesson, we learned what is happening during synaptic transmission: the communication process among neurons in a healthy, non-addicted brain. Here's what is happening in an addicted brain.

The best way to illustrate this process is to begin with a brain addicted to cocaine. When an individual uses cocaine, it activates the VTA, stimulating the production

---

[22] Dopamine transporter blocked by cocaine. https://www.drugabuse.gov/publications/research-reports/cocaine/how-does-cocaine-produce-its-effects

[23] Ken Ashwell, *The Brain Book: Development, Function, Disorder, Health* (Buffalo: Firefly Books Ltd., 2012), 292.

of dopamine.[24] However, with cocaine on board, the cocaine binds to the dopamine transport system and blocks the reuptake process. As a result, dopamine floods the synaptic gap and over stimulates the receiving neuron.

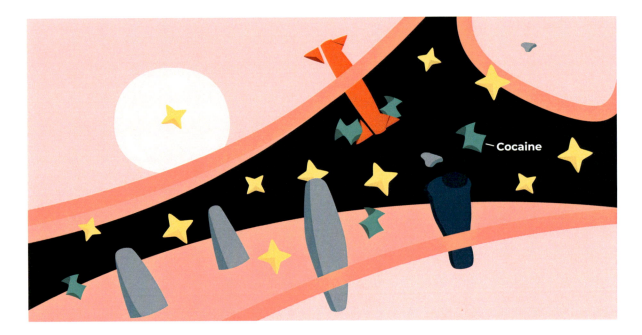

What is most fascinating about this process is that **the brain registers all pleasure the same way, regardless of its origin.**[25] Whether we derive pleasure from shopping, a substance, a sexual encounter, or an accomplishment, the brain responds the same way. In fact, the brain doesn't discriminate based on the source—it will continue to produce dopamine in response to the stimulation of the VTA.

So what is happening in the brain if cocaine is not the issue but a behavior is the issue? What is blocking the reuptake of dopamine? This is an excellent question!

Based on research from the University of Florida, scientists liken the dopamine transport system to a very powerful and efficient "vacuum cleaner."[26] In a healthy brain, when dopamine is released in response to a pleasurable action, dopamine is eventually swept back into the sending cell via the dopamine transport system, returning the brain to a less-stimulated state. Our brain is all about balance. When the dopamine transport system is out of balance—unable to keep up with excessive amounts of dopamine in the system—problems occur.

---

[24] Ken Ashwell, *The Brain Book*, 301-303.

[25] Harvard Mental Health, *Understanding Addiction: How Addiction Hijacks the Brain*. Harvard Health Publications. https://www.helpguide.org/harvard/how-addiction-hijacks-the-brain.htm.

[26] University of Florida. (2016, January 25). Researchers uncover how dopamine transports within the brain. ScienceDaily. www.sciencedaily.com/releases/2016/01/160125184333.htm.

A non-substance addiction is considered a behavioral or process addiction: the compulsion to continually engage in a behavior despite the negative consequences.[27] When it comes to addictive behaviors, a person can find themselves becoming addicted to love, sex, food, shopping, relationships, gaming, and even social media. The brain can become addicted to these behaviors the same way it becomes addicted to a substance.

Consider the difference between substance addiction and process addiction. In most cases, it's easier to see the effects a substance has on a person's behaviors. When it comes to many process addictions, they are easier to hide. Very few people see the effects of sexual addiction in the addict.

✚ What destructive effects have you noticed in your husband (lying, minimizing, gaslighting, refusing to get help, blaming you rather than taking responsibility for his actions, avoiding normal day-to-day responsibilities, and/or isolating)?

This is how a sexually addicted brain is being hijacked. The brain is creating the neurotransmitter, dopamine, that it's addicted to. And what often makes matters worse is how tolerance develops over time.

27 American Addiction Centers (2018). Retrieved from https://americanaddictioncenters.org/behavioral-addictions.

Tolerance
PROGRESSIVE DRUG TOLERANCE

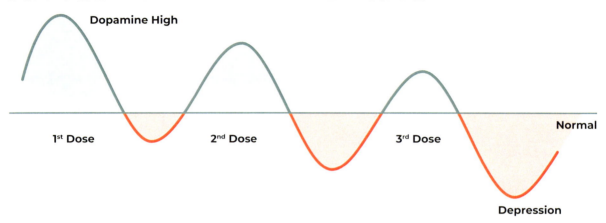

Typically, when our reward system is naturally stimulated through the pleasures of our everyday lives, our brain functions accordingly. However, when we artificially increase the stimulation of dopamine through substance use or behaviors, flooding the brain with excess amounts of dopamine, the brain responds by producing less dopamine.[28] The brain recognizes when something is not right in its chemical makeup and makes adjustments to bring everything back into balance. Over time, the substance or behavior yields less pleasure, requiring an increased dosage of the substance or an escalation in the behavior to achieve the same dopamine high.

When it comes to developing **tolerance**, here's what we need to remember: **an increase in stimuli—the substance or behavior used to make us feel better—decreases the effect it has in the brain.**

This is also one of the main reasons why it is so difficult to stop using a substance or engaging in unhealthy behaviors. The downside of a dopamine high is often followed by anxiety and depression[29]—anxiety because we're now faced with living life without the protection of our addiction, and depression because our brain has decreased its dopamine production.

As a partner, before you discovered his hidden sexual behaviors, you may have noticed times in which your husband didn't seem as satisfied or even capable of regular sexual intimacy. Perhaps he pressured you to do things that seemed immoral or counter to your values or wishes.

---

28 Harvard Mental Health, Understanding Addiction: How Addiction Hijacks the Brain. Harvard Health Publications. https://www.helpguide.org/harvard/how-addiction-hijacks-the-brain.htm.

29 Ken Ashwell, *The Brain Book: Development, Function, Disorder, Health* (Buffalo: Firefly Books Ltd., 2012), 251.

✝ Now that you have learned about his need to increase the stimuli (of his compulsive sexual behaviors) so he can get his high, what kind of emotions does this create in you? Write down your thoughts and feelings about what you have experienced in your sexual relationship with the addict.

_____

_____

_____

_____

_____

_____

_____

_____

_____

_____

_____

For many people who struggle with compulsive sexual behaviors, this Scripture makes so much sense.

> I decide to do good, but I don't really do it; I decide not to do bad, but then I do it anyway.
>
> ROMANS 7:19B (MSG)

This illustrates the internal battle of someone stuck in sexual brokenness. They don't want to do what they are doing. They want to stop. They've tried to stop, many times. But their hijacked brain keeps pulling them back to the behaviors that are familiar and have become part of their automatic response to pain.

So is there any hope for someone trapped in compulsive sexual behaviors?

> Do not conform to the pattern of this world, but be transformed by the renewing of your mind. Then you will be able to test and approve what God's will is—his good, pleasing and perfect will.
>
> ROMANS 12:2 (NIV)

For many men who struggle with sexual brokenness, being part of a Pure Desire group and doing the weekly work helps to facilitate the process of renewing the mind. For the first time, maybe ever, they will face the pain they've spent years running from. They will be given the support and tools they need to re-engage their prefrontal cortex. They will experience handwriting their assignments, which is intentional: research has shown that the physical process of handwriting, instead of typing on a computer, engages the brain.[30] Much like adjusting the lens of a telescope, handwriting has a refining element, enhancing mental change.

✚ **Describe in your own words what you have learned about how the brain is changed through compulsive sexual behaviors.**

✚ **How does learning about an addicted and hijacked brain help you make sense of your husband's behaviors?**

[30] Norman Doidge, *The Brain That Changes Itself* (New York, New York: Penguin Group, 2007), 38.

This information is not intended to excuse, minimize, or justify your husband's behaviors. What he did was wrong. How he hurt you was wrong. Providing this information is for you. So you can make informed decisions about your healing and your future.

For those partners who choose to stay in the relationship, there is hope for your husband's recovery and freedom. These two commitments have made the difference for so many men who struggled with sexual brokenness and have chosen to work on their healing through a men's recovery group.[31]

#1 A COMMITMENT TO HARD WORK AND HONESTY.

Both these areas tend to be foreign territory for those who struggle with sexual brokenness. They may be hard working and honest in many areas of their lives, but with their sexuality, this hasn't been there for a long time. The hard work needed to find healing and freedom will be difficult because the addict will not be in control, which is where honesty comes in. If they are in a Pure Desire recovery group, it will become a safe place where they can test their ability to be honest. Being able to fully trust the other men in their group will be foundational for their recovery.

#2 A COMMITMENT TO TAKE UP THE SWORD OF THE SPIRIT IN THEIR LIFE.

In Paul's description of the warrior God has designed your husband to become, he makes a critical observation:

> *Take the helmet of salvation and the sword of the Spirit,*
> *which is the word of God.*
>
> EPHESIANS 6:17 (NIV)

For true healing and transformation to take place, your husband needs God's Word to be active in his life. He needs the Holy Spirit to speak truth into his life from the Word of God. This is how he will begin to experience a renewed mind, a changed heart, and lifelong freedom.

---

[31] Ted Roberts, *Seven Pillars of Freedom* (Gresham: Pure Desire Ministries International, 2009), 235.

✚ If your husband is a Christ follower. why would these two commitments be important for him to make?

_____

_____

_____

_____

_____

_____

_____

_____

_____

✚ How would these two commitments help build trust between you and your husband?

_____

_____

_____

_____

_____

_____

_____

_____

_____

✝ Regardless of where you are on this journey—married, separated, or divorced—write out a prayer for yourself: asking God to give you strength to find healing from betrayal, discernment when it comes to navigating this relationship, and peace during this process.

How Did He Get This Way ?

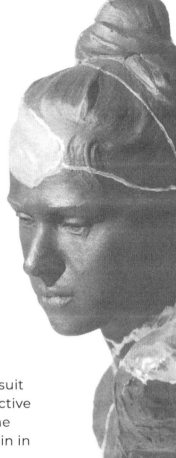

Sexual brokenness causes a person to become fully absorbed in the pursuit of sex, usually at any cost. It is normal for most people to notice an attractive person. But for the sex addict, fantasy and sexual obsession have become primary coping strategies for dealing with stress and medicating the pain in their lives.

THE CYCLONE OF ADDICTION

Many of the factors that contribute to compulsive sexual behavior remain undetected for years. However, as the addict's pain increases, relationships strain, and unresolved trauma continues to show up in their daily lives, they begin to feel the storm building. Much like a cyclone that leaves a trail of destruction in its wake, so it is with compulsive sexual behaviors.

For a cyclone to form, there must be several things present in the environment: air temperature, wind speed, the meeting of a hot and cold front, and more. All of these factors must be present or a cyclone will not form.

This is also true in The Cyclone of Addiction. A number of factors must be present that contribute to an addict's behaviors. Unless they deal with the underlying issues, the storm will continue to build and become uncontainable. But as they work to heal these areas of their lives, they will see The Cyclone of Addiction dissipate and lose its power.

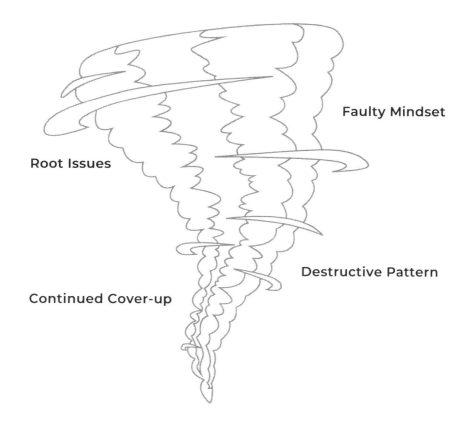

Faulty Mindset

Root Issues

Destructive Pattern

Continued Cover-up

As you look at The Cyclone of Addiction diagram, you can see that there are four elements contributing to this addictive lifestyle: Root Issues, a Faulty Mindset, Destructive Patterns, and the Continued Cover-Up.

The Root Issues is where it all started. Sexual brokenness can start from one or all three of the following elements:

- Family of origin dysfunction
- Early abuse and personal trauma
- Growing up in an addictive society

How can these Root Issues produce sexual brokenness? First, all family systems are dysfunctional to some degree. We all make mistakes and, like Adam and Eve, we all have a sin nature. Early negative family experiences often cause a child to feel shame that can linger into adulthood. Many people think that shame and guilt are basically the same type of emotion, but they are quite different. Guilt says, "I did something wrong." Shame says, "There is something wrong with me; I am defective." Shame is at the core of every addiction. For example, if a child feels they can never measure up, never have control in their lives, and never receives unconditional love, sexual activity can be a way of soothing their pain and fear.

Second, personal trauma, which could be caused by abuse, can lead to a desire to avoid the pain by escaping into a sexual world. Statistically, 97% of sexual addicts have been emotionally abused, 72% physically abused, and 81% sexually abused.[32] There is a saying in recovery groups: **Discover the trauma and you will understand the addiction.**

Third, our culture can impact a person through peer pressure and make them vulnerable to sexual brokenness. The disposition of a family (the environment in which a person is raised)—especially where alcohol abuse and inappropriate sexual behaviors are involved—can literally cause a neurochemical change in the brain that sets up individuals to be predisposed to addictive behavior.[33]

✚ From what you know about your husband, what Root Issues have contributed to his compulsive sexual behaviors ?

_____

_____

_____

_____

_____

Shame then moves the addict from struggling with Root Issues to battling a **Faulty Mindset** in which control, entitlement, escape from reality, and pleasure-seeking begins to inundate many areas of their life. The underlying thoughts and feelings they are struggling with include some or all of the following:

- Core beliefs of unworthiness/shame
- Discomfort with feeling alone
- False concept of need for sex

Many men experienced these elements from an early age. Feeling unworthy and alone led them to use sex as a means of numbing their emotional pain. They continue using compulsive sexual behavior to avoid the pain when feeling stressed. The enemy plays off these feelings of worthlessness and wants the addict to believe he is the only one who has this struggle and it is because he is defective—something is wrong with him. Many addicts were raised in a home where messages regarding sexual feelings and behaviors were negatively communicated and viewed as wrong. These attitudes only increased the shame.

---

[32] Patrick Carnes, _Don't Call It Love: Recovery From Sexual Addiction_ (New York: Bantam Books, 1991), 104.

[33] National Institute on Drug Abuse, _Drugs, Brains, and Behavior: The Science of Addiction_, NIH Pub No. 14-5605, July 2014.

The pain of the Root Issues and a Faulty Mindset can easily lead to the next step, which is **Destructive Patterns.**

- Preoccupation
- Ritualization
- Compulsion
- Despair

The first phase, **Preoccupation**, is a focus on sexual thoughts and fantasies that brings a mood altering "high" without actually acting out. Fantasy can be a means of avoiding the pain of the present reality or past hurts from childhood. Once a certain level of fantasy dominates an addict's thinking, it is difficult for the addict to shut down the process. Everyday responsibilities such as work, deadlines, and family can rapidly diminish in importance as the obsession takes control. **Most of the addict's time in this first phase is spent in fantasy.**[34]

✚ From your observations, how has your husband's addiction and/or fantasy life affected his ability to meet deadlines, have time for family, and be present in the moment?

Many women have observed that procrastination, passivity, and isolation are usually an indication that their husband is struggling with his addiction.

---

[34] Ted Roberts, *For Men Only* (Gresham: East Hill Church, 1993), 26-27.

✚ **Can you relate to any of these indicators? What effects have they had on you and the family?**

Ritualization becomes the next phase where a lot of time is spent preparing to act out sexually. The ritual phase might include:

- Planning times late at night to be on the computer
- Isolating on the phone or tablet
- Driving by the adult bookstore or strip clubs
- Cruising the street looking for prostitutes
- Going to singles or gay bars
- Renting X-rated DVDs or viewing X-rated websites

Ritualization is frequently used to bring comfort in times of crisis or conflict. Rituals can be reactive in nature. For example, an addict may pick a fight with his wife, and then act out sexually in self-righteous anger. He may also make inappropriate sexual overtures to his wife, thus setting up a rejection scenario that gives him the sense of justifying his sexual behaviors. Living a life of stress and overload can also send him into one crisis after another.

✚ **You may or may not be aware of your husband's rituals, but can you identify with any of the reactive behaviors? Explain.**

Once the ritual begins, he will feel the **Compulsion** to act out. He then feels guilt and shame and vows to never do it again.

Then he moves into the next phase of **Despair**. Sexual addiction is much like food addiction in that 72% of sex addicts use what is called a "binge and purge" cycle.[35] They are sexually compulsive and act out, and then they sexually starve themselves because of the shame. The behavior can go to extremes through either total control or no control. Romans 7 gives us insight into this situation:

> I don't understand myself at all, for I really want to do what is right [sexual health], but I can't. I do what I don't want to [ritual]—what I hate.
>
> ROMANS 7:15 (TLB)

The addict's ability to manage the stress of life is underdeveloped. As soon as the next stressor comes along and feels unmanageable, he will numb out by fantasizing and the cycle begins again.

Going back to The Cyclone of Addition, we see that the **Continued Cover-Up** consists of:

- Denial
- Rationalizing
- Minimizing
- Delusion
- Blaming others

The addict uses each of these as a coping mechanism to justify living a double life. Any or all of these coping behaviors allows the addict to compartmentalize his life and live in two worlds.

The Continued Cover-Up produces distorted thinking such as, "I am not hurting anyone," "I am so stressed, I need a distraction," or "I had such a bad day, I am entitled to some relief." These distorted thoughts fill his mind and he begins to justify his behavior so he can continue in his compulsive sexual behaviors. He begins believing these lies to the point of thinking they are his reality.

This explanation is not meant to excuse, minimize, or justify the addict's behavior. This information is meant to empower you with a look into the soul of the addict.

---

[35] Patrick Carnes, "Sexual Addiction and Compulsion: Recognition, Treatment & Recovery," *CNS Spectrums 5*, no. 10 (October 2000): 63-72.

✚ Summarize what you have learned about The Cyclone of Addiction and how you think your husband might fit into the different areas: Root Issues; a Faulty Mindset; Destructive Patterns; and the Continued Cover-Up.

How Will I Know If He's Changing ?

We've talked about how an addict's faulty mindset and their feelings of worthlessness are key issues driving the behaviors. Shame is at the core of their behaviors; hiding this shame becomes a means of survival, a way to deaden and escape pain. It also becomes a means of filling the hole of emotional wounds left by a lack of safety and nurturing in their childhood.

Most men who struggle are able to control their behaviors for periods of time, but in reality, they are using the Continued Cover-Up. When stress, pain, or old messages of worthlessness begin haunting him, he will often revert back to acting out.

Picture their life as one of those "whack-a-mole" games, where he is trying to hit everything that pops up with a mallet. When he has the energy to control his addictive behaviors, he is ACTING IN; in other words, he is trying hard to keep everything under control. But when the pain level rises and he can no longer control his behavior, he will ACT OUT. For many who struggle, the cycle vacillates from control (acting in) to keep up the false image, then to out-of-control (acting out) to release the pressure of trying to measure up.

Ninety-two percent of addicts feel as though they are living in these two extremes.[36] How can they stop the pendulum's swing from chaotic, out-of-control behavior, to controlled behavior that is rigid and emotionally closed down?[37]

---

[36] Patrick Carnes, *Don't Call It Love: Recovery From Sexual Addiction* (New York: Bantam Books, 1991), 105.

[37] Ted Roberts and Diane Roberts, *Hope for Men* (Gresham: Pure Desire Ministries International, 2012), 31.

THE CONTINUUM OF SEXUALITY[38]

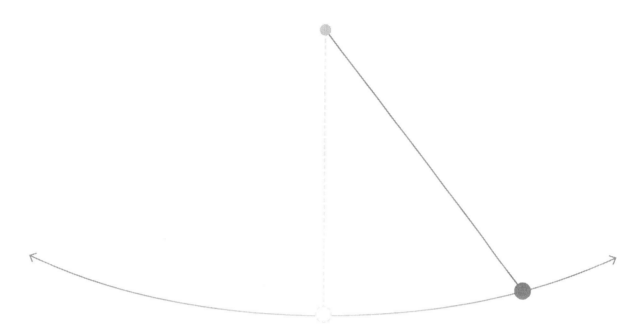

Sexual Anorexia/ Acting In	Sexual Health	Sexual Addiction/ Acting Out
Rigid	Structure	Chaotic
Excessive	Boundaries	Collapse
Isolation	Intimacy	Emotionally Absent
Depression	Expressing Needs	Excess
Fear	Sharing Needs	Anger
Obsessive	Taking Responsibility	Defiant

[38] Adapted from International Institute for Trauma and Addiction Professionals CSAT Certification Training Day Two: Module One

This could include behaviors such as:

- The addict is sexually anorexic with his wife but sexually acts out with porn, affairs, and prostitutes.
- After having an affair, the addict abstains from having any contact with his affair partner but then begins to overwork.
- The addict relapses with porn and feels guilty; he abstains from porn but begins compulsively playing video games.

Healthy balanced behaviors include:

- Structure
- Boundaries
- Intimacy
- Expressing needs
- Sharing needs/feelings
- Taking responsibility

Under the pendulum labeled "Sexual Health," the skills above are also listed. What skills and behaviors would your spouse need to learn and develop for the pendulum of acting in and acting out to stop?

✚ Put a check mark next to all that apply and explain why they are important to you.

In order to get healthy, most men began to realize that trying harder never works. The key is discovering the core of the shame and facing it. Ultimately, they will find greater healing when they begin to understand where the worthless messages come from and that God looks past the behavior to see and love him for who he is.

A partner can easily be deceived by her husband's behaviors when he is trying hard to be in control. She may be fooled by his "acting in" behaviors and think her husband is getting better.

This is why it's important for you to have this information. So you know the truth about his motivations and behaviors. It will help you accurately assess his behaviors and equip you to address issues that make you feel unsafe.

What can help interrupt the acting in and acting out cycle? How can you tell if he's changing and moving toward health? One of the main indicators is seeing your husband incorporate healthy structures and boundaries in his life.

Examples of healthy structures and boundaries for him:

- Weekly participation in a recovery group, such as Seven Pillars of Freedom
- Completing recovery homework on a consistent basis
- Regular accountability that includes phone calls each week to accountability partners
- Accountability software on all his electronic devices (even downgrading to a phone without internet access if needed)
- Making family and his relationship with God a priority
- Being mentally and emotionally present, working on intimacy and connectedness
- Taking responsibility for his actions
- Proactively using recovery tools and self-care for developing healthy habits
- Knowing each day where he is on the FASTER Scale
- No contact with the person or persons with whom he has been sexual
- Possibly a polygraph test every three to six months if deep trust issues exist

Some or all of these behaviors may be incorporated in your Safety Action Plan.

The list of what a healthy lifestyle looks like is probably foreign to most men who struggle with compulsive sexual behaviors. He doesn't know how to establish boundaries or have structure, and rarely has an understanding of what a healthy relationship looks like. For his recovery, he will need a group of men, and possibly a counselor, who can help him begin to feel comfortable sharing real feelings, taking responsibility, learning discernment about his behaviors, and discovering what painful events from his past have contributed to his addictive behavior.

✝ **Think about the last time your husband was "acting in"-controlling his addictive behaviors. List the behaviors you noticed.**

✝ Make a list of the past/childhood painful events you think contribute to your husband's compulsive sexual behaviors. What untreated pain/trauma is driving his behaviors?

_____

_____

_____

_____

_____

_____

_____

_____

_____

_____

_____

_____

_____

_____

For your husband, it is likely these painful past experiences and lies he believes about himself have caused him to live a double life. Most men find freedom when they begin to face their fears and unpack the painful experiences from their past. Most men have been running from their pain and have tried to stay ahead of the avalanche by acting out, lying, gaslighting, manipulating, and medicating their pain. Real healing begins when they stop running and start to face the fears and lies. Rather than his behaviors swinging from control to out-of-control extremes, the addict will begin to move into a place of trusting God.

Galatians gives us the key:

> Does the God who lavishly provides you with his own presence, his Holy Spirit, working things in your lives you could never do for yourselves, does he do these things because of your strenuous moral striving or because you trust him to do them in you?
>
> GALATIANS 3:5 (MSG)

Moving into a healthy place will require the addict to trust God in new ways. Sharing his needs and real feelings requires a vulnerability that he has never had in his life. One of his greatest fears is that he will reveal his true self and be rejected. But working through these fears will become a steady piece of his recovery journey.

Because it takes time to see real progress in recovery, most counselors and experts recommend the betrayed partner not make any major decisions (such as divorce) for a year. It usually takes this long to see if the addict is moving toward a place of true sobriety in his recovery process. Remember, he likely has been struggling with this for years and it will take time for him to change direction and experience some victory.

✚ After learning more about the origins of compulsive sexual behaviors and how past pain and trauma drive an addict's behaviors, how do you feel? What thoughts and feelings are you experiencing right now?

Note: If you are feeling triggered by any of the lesson content or this healing process, and want to pursue professional help, please contact Pure Desire at 503-489-0230 or visit **puredesire.org/counseling**.

6

What is the Role of Full Disclosure, Intensives, and Counseling ?

Understanding Disclosure

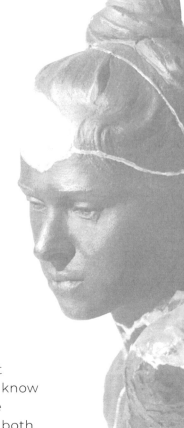

In this lesson, we want to explore the difficulty of disclosure and how it impacts the family. Since you are processing this material, you already know some or all of what your husband has been involved in. If there is more disclosure and he is in a men's recovery group, it's recommended that both you and your husband have the support of your counselor and/or group leader to process the full disclosure. At any point, you can contact Pure Desire to schedule Full Disclosure Counseling and have a clinical team walk through this process with you.[1]

 Twenty years of deception can be divulged in fifteen minutes, leaving the wife shell-shocked, confused, and loaded with unwanted shrapnel in her skin. These mishandled admissions are more common than we'd like to think. They can be incomplete, ill-timed, one-sided surprises that catch us off guard.[2]

There are three types of disclosure: forced disclosure, staggered disclosure, and full disclosure.

---

[1] For more information about Pure Desire's Full Disclosure Counseling, call 503-489-0230 or visit puredesire.org/program-overview.

[2] Sheri Keffer, *Intimate Deception: Healing the Wounds of Sexual Betrayal* (Grand Rapids: Revell Books, 2018), 249.

In some cases, an immediate disclosure is necessary. This is referred to as **forced disclosure**. Such cases include when a spouse has been caught in the act, when illegal activity has occurred, when sexual activity involves other people and potential STDs/STIs, or when the betrayed partner feels unable to move forward in spite of other support in place (e.g., part of a Pure Desire group).

Staggered disclosure happens when bits and pieces of the addict's behaviors are revealed or discovered, which can contribute to the trauma experienced by the partner. Preventing staggered disclosure is an important part of this process.

One study found that:

...75% of the women studied uncovered or discovered evidence of compulsive or addictive sexual behaviors themselves, as opposed to a planned disclosure or confession on the part of their husbands. While this was consistent with previous research, this result illustrated the degree of suddenness or surprise surrounding the disclosure episode that may contribute to the traumatic nature of disclosure.[3]

✚ Have you experienced any form of forced or staggered disclosure? Explain.

✚ If so, how did it affect you?

---

[3] Barbara Steffens and Robyn Rennie, "The Traumatic Nature of Disclosure for Wives of Sexual Addicts," *Sexual Addiction & Compulsivity*, 13:247-267, 2006.

The disclosure process is a critical, yet challenging aspect of this healing journey. **Full disclosure** is defined as a full, fact-based reporting of the addict's sexual history and is usually recommended after six months of focused recovery work. When possible, disclosure should be done with a Certified Sex Addiction Therapist (CSAT) or Pastoral Sex Addiction Professional Supervisor (PSAP-S). If disclosure is done incorrectly, it can do much more harm to the partner.

It is important for you to learn about the disclosure process and what healthy disclosure looks like. This can also be quite challenging, because you may be early in your healing journey and disclosure for you might still be several months away. Do your best to trust the process, knowing that it is the healthiest approach for both you and your husband.

✚ At this point in your journey, how much of his addiction are you aware of? Describe why you think the extent might be greater than what you know now.

✚ What do you think and feel about waiting for a future time for him to give you a full disclosure (presuming he is diligently working on his recovery in a Seven Pillars of Freedom group)?

Although the full disclosure process often happens after six months of focused recovery work, it is critical to the healing process that the addict learns to be transparent while working toward sobriety. When relapse(s) occurs during the recovery process, it should be disclosed to group members and their partner. Immediately after relapse occurs, your Safety Action Plan should be implemented.

During recovery, your spouse will learn to live an honest lifestyle, break isolation, relate behaviors to consequences, and give the people who they have hurt the respect and dignity to make informed choices. This is less likely to happen if your spouse is working on recovery, but still keeping secrets.

The following is an outline of important steps for the betrayed partner and addict spouse to take leading up to, during, and after full disclosure has occurred.

STEPS FOR THE BETRAYED PARTNER

Write out questions that are needed to establish truth, understanding, and forward motion in your healing. Keep in mind that restoration and healing should be the driving force behind these questions. Avoid questions that may hinder your healing and only cause you more pain. Examples of commonly asked questions are:

- In what ways have you lied about or hidden behaviors from me?
- What are the addictive behaviors you are/were involved with?
- What are the time frames of these behaviors?
  - ▷ What was the frequency and duration?
- Has your behavior involved another person/other people?
  - ▷ How many other partners were there?
  - ▷ What were the places and locations of these encounters?
  - ▷ Do I know any of the people you were sexually involved with?
  - ▷ Have you cut off all contact with anyone you have acted out with?
- Has any of your sexual acting out included same-sex relationships or behaviors?

Share these questions with your husband before the disclosure, so he has time to formulate honest, thorough answers. These may be shared through your counselor, who is familiar with the disclosure process, or group leader. This person might suggest omitting certain questions to help you avoid questions that are overly detailed or hold more potential for pain than healing.

It is recommended that full disclosure is done with a professional counselor, who is trained and experienced in the disclosure process. Including any other outside people in the disclosure process should always be at the choosing and comfort level of the betrayed partner.

STEPS FOR THE ADDICTED SPOUSE

Your spouse will write out his full sexual history. The following list provides details of common information revealed during disclosure.[4]

- Include the time frame when referring to each incident where he acted out and how many times incidents happened during that time frame.
- Include sex acts that don't involve a physical act, such as flirting or planning to act out.
- Include financial information.
- Include health issues or health risks such as exposure to STDs.
- Acknowledge if this involves someone else who their wife may know or run into.
- Refer to their wife in the second person (I betrayed YOU when...).
- Stick with information sharing; they are not to justify any of their addictive behavior.

Before sharing with their spouse, they will share this written disclosure with their counselor who is familiar and experienced with the disclosure process and/or group leader.

Pure Desire offers full disclosure counseling; for more information, visit **puredesire.org/program-overview**. Counseling support for partners is also available through APSATS (The Association of Partners of Sex Addicts Trauma Specialists); for more information, visit **www.apsats.org**.

Given an appropriate amount of time following disclosure, both the betrayed partner and addict spouse should work together to find a time for an honest conversation to emotionally process the disclosure. If you choose to do this, it may be helpful to include your counselor or group leader in this follow-up conversation.

 Disclosure is not the end of talking about your sexual history... it's the beginning...if your relationship is going to last.[5]

---

[4] Ted Roberts, *Seven Pillars of Freedom* (Gresham: Pure Desire Ministries International, 2009), 201.

[5] Barbara Steffens, *Disclosure Trauma*, Multidimensional Partner Trauma Model Training, Day 2, June 12, 2021, The Association of Partners of Sex Addicts Trauma Specialists (APSATS).

IS DISCLOSURE THE RIGHT THING TO DO?

Many couples wonder if disclosure is the right thing to do. During this research, addicts and their partners were asked two questions about disclosure:[6]

- "Initially, how did you feel at the time about the disclosure?"
- "Looking back now at the disclosure, how do you feel about it now?"

For the sex addict, only 58% initially felt disclosure was the right thing to do. Looking back, 96% of sex addicts felt it was the right thing to do.

For the partners, 81% initially felt disclosure was the right thing to do. Looking back, 93% of partners felt it was the right thing to do.

After going through the disclosure process, both the addict (96%) and their partner (93%) felt that disclosure was the right thing to do.

In the midst of everything you're going through, it can be difficult to weigh the pros and cons of disclosure. In her book, *Intimate Deception*, Dr. Sheri Keffer highlights some of the benefits and risks of disclosure.[7]

Benefits

- Restored truth
- Confrontation of deception
- Hope for a future relationship
- Betraying spouse is able to get free from their secrets and shame
- Betrayed spouse is empowered to make informed decisions about the future

Risks

- Increased shame and guilt
- Temporary separations or divorce
- Financial, legal, or professional consequences
- Changes in family function, including limited access to children
- Loss of trust; the relationship may get worse before it gets better

---

[6] Jennifer Schneider, Deborah Corley, and Richard Irons, "Surviving Disclosure of Infidelity: Results of an International Survey of 164 Recovering Sex Addicts and Partners," *Sexual Addiction & Compulsivity*, 5:189-217, 1998.

[7] Sheri Keffer, *Intimate Deception: Healing the Wounds of Sexual Betrayal* (Grand Rapids: Revell Books, 2018), 254.

While the disclosure process can be tough, when done well, it can be an instrumental healing tool. Here are a few additional things to consider when it comes to disclosure.[8]

- A betrayed partner cannot heal until they know what they need to heal from.
  - ▷ She is often haunted by unanswered questions, doubts, and fears.
  - ▷ Her fears are often worse than reality.
- Disclosure helps to build a strong foundation for the relationship.
  - ▷ Secrets create barriers to intimacy.
- Disclosure challenges dysfunctional core beliefs for both the partner and the addict.
  - ▷ Helps the partner recognize the addiction was there before her; it's not about her.
- Disclosure removes the power of secrets.
  - ▷ Secrets fuel shame → Shame fuels relapse.

✚ **When considering the previously mentioned benefits and risks involved in disclosure, which of these resonate with you?**

---

[8] Barbara Steffens, *Disclosure Trauma*, Multidimensional Partner Trauma Model Training, Day 2, June 12, 2021, The Association of Partners of Sex Addicts Trauma Specialists (APSATS).

+ Based on your specific situation, are there any other benefits and/or risks you are concerned about?

_____
_____
_____
_____
_____
_____
_____
_____
_____
_____

THE PURPOSE OF A POLYGRAPH

During the disclosure process, many experts and professionals who work in this environment have found it helpful to use a polygraph test.

Dr. Milton Magness, an expert who works with sex addicts and regularly uses polygraphs, stated:

Because of the core belief of sex addicts that people will not love me as I am, I believe it is virtually impossible to get a complete disclosure without a polygraph exam to verify that the disclosure is not just a sanitized version of events the sex addict hopes his partner will forgive. Unless the whole truth is told, the sex addict does not have the opportunity to get free from his behaviors. And unless the addict can get honest with his partner, they do not have the opportunity of ever restoring trust in the relationship.[9]

In most cases, the addict spouse will work with a counselor to write out a full, fact-based disclosure that is thorough and honest. Then they will take a polygraph test to ensure the truthfulness of the disclosure.

---

[9] Sheri Keffer, _Intimate Deception: Healing the Wounds of Sexual Betrayal_ (Grand Rapids: Revell Books, 2018), 258.

It is important to understand what a polygraph test can and cannot do.[10]

- A polygraph should not focus on failing someone, but should help a person establish truthfulness.
- A polygraph deals with absolutes; questions that yield a yes/no answer.
- A polygraph is not helpful when answering complex questions about thoughts, feelings, and intentions.
- A polygraph is intended to verify several clear and direct questions, such as, "Is what you have written in this disclosure true?"

Once the truthfulness of the disclosure is verified, the disclosure between the addict spouse and the betrayed partner will take place.

Dr. Magness further explains:

The idea of having a polygraph examination following a disclosure may bring hope to the spouses of sexual addicts, because they realize that with its use they can finally believe they have gotten the whole truth and not have to imagine and worry about what else in which their partners may be involved. Without a polygraph exam, the partner has no assurance that he or she is hearing the complete truth.[11]

Using a polygraph may not be the process for every couple, but knowing the options surrounding disclosure helps a betrayed partner make informed decisions. More information about a polygraph test can be found in the appendix on page 326.

✚ How would using a polygraph test help in your current situation?

---

[10] Keffer, *Intimate Deception*, 258.

[11] Barbara Steffens and Marsha Means, *Your Sexually Addicted Spouse: How Partners Can Cope and Heal* (Far Hills: New Horizon Press, 2009), 115.

✚ You and your husband may be working toward disclosure. How would you define where you are in this process?

1 **2** **3** **4** **5**

No Disclosure   Full Disclosure

✚ What are some things you can do to prepare yourself if more disclosure will need to take place?

_____
_____
_____
_____
_____
_____
_____
_____
_____
_____
_____
_____
_____
_____
_____
_____
_____
_____
_____

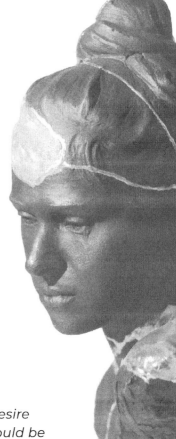

I Need Help Now

Early in our marriage, my husband had confessed to previous struggles with pornography, but claimed he no longer struggled. So when Pure Desire brought a two-day conference to our church, my husband thought it would be great for us to attend, so we could be a part of helping others who struggle.

After the first night of the conference, on our way to pick up our two-year-old son, my husband was a bit reserved. He made comments like, "Wow, it's so sad for people who are caught up in sex addiction..." and "I wonder if people are ever fully healed from sex addiction?" At the time, I didn't think much of it.

The next day of the conference included several different sessions with breaks in between sessions. I'm not sure what happened to my husband during the initial session, but during that first break, he started confessing to me small details about his current porn use. He said things like, "I'm sorry I didn't tell you, but I look at porn every few months...it's not that often..." I was shocked! When does he do this? We spend so much time together and as a family. We have a great relationship! Or so I thought.

By the lunch break, my husband was confessing more than my ears could hear: porn and masturbation on a regular basis, and even a short affair early in our marriage. And yet, he kept saying, "But I love you!" I couldn't stop crying. My mind was racing. I told him I didn't want to hear any more of this today, but it's like he couldn't stop himself.

Although I was eight months pregnant with our second child, by the end of the conference, all I wanted was a divorce. I didn't even know the whole story, but I didn't care. I was so devastated and hurt, I only wanted to get away from this person who said he loved me. At that point, I was pretty sure our marriage wouldn't make it.

MARTINA

When disclosure happens and a partner is completely unaware of her husband's struggle, this can immediately throw the relationship into crisis. If there is any hope for the relationship to survive, they may need an intensive form of therapy.

More traditional types of therapy or counseling happen over long periods of time. Typically, a person will meet with a counselor for an hour, once every week or two, for an extended period of time.[12] They often meet over the course of a year or more. With this type of therapy, it may take a couple weeks to a month to schedule an initial appointment with a counselor. And for most people who are not in crisis, they are okay with this waiting period.

An intensive form of therapy is much different. It is a more in-depth and focused approach that takes place over a short period of time. So instead of meeting with the counselor for an hour every week, they meet with a counselor (or are involved in a clinical program) for eight hours each day, over a period of several days. It is more of a fast track form of therapy that is specifically designed to help individuals or couples who are in immediate crisis.

While many intensive programs are intended to help resolve or deescalate crisis situations, they are not meant to replace the extensive healing and recovery that happens through long-term counseling programs. For this reason, Pure Desire offers counseling programs for partners and couples who want to create sustainable healing and recovery.

Intensive Programs

There are several types of intensive programs for partners who have experienced betrayal trauma, for those who struggle with compulsive sexual behaviors, and for couples who want to pursue healing and recovery together.

When the initial disclosure or discovery happens, some partners would benefit from an intensive program that focuses specifically on them.[13] This type of program provides a small group environment, where a partner feels safe to share their story with others who have experienced betrayal. Over a short number of days, they receive education about betrayal trauma and the impact of their spouse's hidden sexual behaviors, as well as resources and tools to help during the beginning stages of their healing. This all happens within a supportive community of trained professionals.

---

[12] Pure Desire offers a clinical program that works with couples, counseling them together in tandem with their individual group experience. This clinical approach is most successful when working with couples in the beginning stages of their healing and recovery journey.

[13] Banyan Therapy Group: for more information, visit https://www.banyantherapy.com/intensives/.

There are also similar intensive programs for those who struggle with compulsive sexual behaviors. These intensives often focus on providing a solid foundation for ongoing recovery, as well as education on how their addictive behaviors have impacted others, especially their partner.

Then there are intensive programs for couples. This includes intensives for those in crisis, who need immediate help, and for those who need other types of intensives throughout their healing and recovery journey.

For example, some couples may benefit from an intensive program that is customized to their specific needs.[14] Or perhaps, a few months into their healing and recovery journey, they may want to take advantage of an intensive disclosure program. Or, for couples who get stuck in their healing and recovery, and need extra help along the way, they may benefit from an intensive program that helps to rebuild aspects of their relationship.

Many intensive programs are developed and run by trained, licensed counselors with years of experience helping couples navigate the fall out of compulsive sexual behaviors and betrayal trauma.

It takes two healthy individuals to build a healthy coupleship, but it's not an automatic process just because both of you are in personal recovery. Couples' healing takes the same focused attention, tools, and commitment as your individual process. The Couples Workshop is the best – quickest, most powerful and cost-effective – way to get a jumpstart on your growth as a couple.[15]

While many intensive programs are private and include only one couple and counselors, there are other programs that facilitate more of a group counseling environment that includes several couples at once.[16] This may be a great option for couples who have done some initial work on their healing and recovery, but continue to experience a higher level of marital distress.

---

[14] Daring Ventures: for more information, visit https://www.daringventures.com/intensives/.

[15] Bethesda Workshops: for more information, visit https://www.bethesdaworkshops.org/workshops/healing-for-couples/.

[16] Hope Restored, Focus on the Family: for more information, visit https://hoperestored.focusonthefamily.com/intensives/what-is-an-intensive/.

✚ Considering Martina's story at the beginning of this lesson, what type of intensive program might benefit her and/or her marriage?

✚ Have you experienced any type of intensive program? If so, explain.?

✚ If you have not experienced any type of intensive program, what thoughts and feelings do you have about participating in an intensive program?

_____

_____

_____

_____

_____

_____

_____

_____

_____

✚ At this point in your healing, how might an intensive program help you and/or your husband, and/or your relationship?

_____

_____

_____

_____

_____

_____

_____

_____

_____

_____

Counseling and Therapy

When partners begin their healing journey, many will join a support group, like this one. Through this experience, they learn they are not alone, feel heard and validated for what they've been through, and are able to significantly move forward in their healing. However, some partners may need additional support through personal counseling or therapy.

Although the terms "counseling" and "therapy" are often used interchangeably, they are different in some aspects.[17] Generally, when a person is in counseling, they tend to focus on one specific problem over a shorter period of time. For example, If a person is struggling with anorexia or bulimia, they would likely see a counselor to help them with their eating disorder. In many cases, this form of counseling would take place on a weekly or biweekly basis, where the counselor and client would work together to resolve the issues surrounding the eating disorder.

Therapy, on the other hand, tends to focus more on the individual and the various issues with which they need help. This may include aspects of stress management, emotional awareness, healthy communication, positive self-talk, establishing boundaries, developing personal goals, and more. Typically, therapy happens over a longer period of time, meeting weekly or biweekly, and works to reshape the individual's perspective of themselves, others, and their world view.

Within the context of counseling and therapy, many counselors will spend several weeks getting to know their client. They will make several assessments based on the client's overall health: behavioral, emotional, physical, relational, and mental health.[18] However, when a person is in crisis, the immediate goals are more focused.

When counselors respond, they are intervening in the crisis. In this intervention, counselors are basically assessing the crisis situation at that moment, stabilizing the person, and assisting in the development of a plan to help them move out of the crisis mode.[19]

Today, when it comes to finding the right type of support, there are many options for partners.

Pure Desire offers Spouse Support Counseling, which is a 12 month program for partners who have experienced betrayal trauma.[20] This program also supports and

---

[17] Jessica Lammers, *Therapy vs. counseling: Is there a difference? Which is right for you?* Ohio State Health & Discovery, March 14, 2022, https://health.osu.edu/health/mental-health/therapy-vs-counseling-is-there-a-difference.

[18] Geri Miller, *Fundamentals of Crisis Counseling* (Hoboken: John Wiley & Sons, Inc., 2012), 3ff.

[19] Geri Miller, *Fundamentals of Crisis Counseling*, 3ff.

[20] For more information, visit puredesire.org/program-overview/.

reinforces the tools partners are learning about during their group experience. Pure Desire also provides podcast episodes and blogs specifically focused on partners who have experienced betrayal trauma.

The Association of Partners of Sex Addicts Trauma Specialists (APSATS) offers counseling and coaching support for partners affected by betrayal trauma.[21] For ongoing guidance and support, APSATS also offers blogs and podcast episodes.

Some organizations offer online courses that will help partners gain a greater understanding of how they have been impacted by the trauma of betrayal.[22] Especially during the early stages of healing, some partners benefit from working at their own pace, learning how betrayal is affecting them, and what steps they can take to start moving forward in their healing.

Any and all of these options might be helpful for partners who want to invest more in themselves and their healing journey.

The first couple days after the conference are a blur. My mind was consumed with everything my husband had confessed. And honestly, I knew there was probably more I didn't know. That week, I canceled various activities I had planned and focused on taking care of my son and myself, since I was a few weeks away from delivery. Since I didn't want to talk about it yet, my husband did his best to be helpful with our son, but stayed away and slept in another room.

What I didn't know at the time was that my husband went to our pastor and confessed everything that happened during the conference. I think he was desperate to save our marriage. Our pastor recommended that we start seeing the counselor on staff and we were able to get an appointment with them the following week.

It has been a challenging six months, but we're still together. We are in counseling with people who are trained in dealing with compulsive sexual behaviors and betrayal trauma. And we are both in groups: I'm in a support group for betrayed partners and he's in a recovery group. Some days, I still wonder if our marriage will make it. Other days, I see small areas of improvement, where I know God is working to soften and heal my heart. While I don't trust my husband yet, I trust God and His ability to do the impossible.

MARTINA

---

[21] The Association of Partners of Sex Addicts Trauma Specialists: for more information, visit https://www.apsats.org/partners.

[22] Bloom for Women, *Healing Trauma From Sexual Betrayal with Dr. Kevin Skinner*: for more information, visit https://bloomforwomen.com/course/healing-from-betrayal-trauma/.

✚ What part(s) of Martina's story do you relate to most?

_____

_____

_____

_____

_____

✚ How has learning about counseling and therapy options impacted you?

_____

_____

_____

_____

_____

✚ What thoughts and feelings do you have about seeking counseling
or therapy for yourself and/or your marriage?

_____

_____

_____

_____

_____

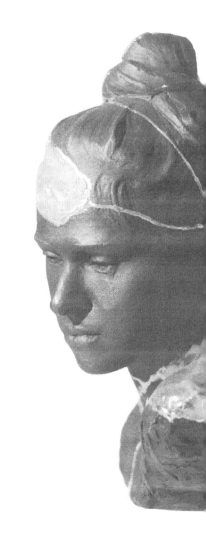

How Will Working On My Own Healing Help Me in the Long Run ?

I learned about my husband's behaviors 15 years into our marriage. I knew something was going on, that there had been a wall between us, but didn't know what was creating it. Although I had noticed the way he flirted with women over the years, and this had been a source of tension in our marriage, I was shocked when I discovered some text messages on his phone to other women. He said he didn't have any physical contact with these women, only a few in-person conversations and text messages. He had lied about this issue for years, so I wasn't sure what to believe.

At the time, my husband said he would do anything to save our marriage and got into a recovery group right away. I didn't want to join a support group for betrayed partners, because this wasn't my issue. It was his! But after a few months of feeling *so angry with him, I realized that a support group might help me process the anger I was feeling.*

After several months of not seeing any real change in my husband's behaviors, I gave him an ultimatum: either we get into counseling to help save our relationship or you can leave today. I'm not going to continue to live this way. I was willing to work on our relationship as long as we continued to move forward.

Within a few weeks, we had started the evaluation process and then began biweekly counseling with a male and female counseling team. It was a lot of work and challenged us in many ways, but I could see small changes in my husband's attitude and behavior. It seemed to be working. But there was one very specific issue that never came up during our counseling sessions. I was trying to trust the process and waiting for this issue to come up, but it never did. It didn't make sense to me: we were preparing for disclosure and had never discussed this one issue that was clearly at the core of my husband's behaviors.

I couldn't take it any more. During the session that was supposed to lead into disclosure, I stopped the session and brought this issue to light. My husband sat there like he didn't know what I was talking about. And it soon became obvious that he had never mentioned this issue to his counselor when they met separately. Right then, my husband and his counselor left the room. When they returned, his counselor said they had more work to do, which ended up postponing disclosure for several weeks.

Later that day, my husband apologized for not mentioning this issue sooner and acknowledged that it was a bigger issue than he wanted to admit. While this was a difficult conversation, it was probably the most honest conversation we'd had in a long time. And during this conversation, the wall between us was gone.

KALANI

✚ **What thoughts and feelings do you have about Kalani's story?**

_____

_____

_____

_____

_____

_____

_____

_____

We have talked about how the healing journey can feel like a two-steps-forward-one-step-back process. Many partners may get to a point where they feel frustrated and unsure if it's working or worth it.

In many ways, this process is like physical therapy. For example, if a person falls and fractures the bones in their leg, the doctors will likely put their leg in a cast or brace to keep it from moving for an extended period of time. During this time, the leg is not being used. It is completely immobilized. And all of this is helping to reduce the pain and protect it from further injury while the bones heal. Although this is one of the best ways to heal the bones, the muscles weaken and even atrophy because of a lack of movement and exercise. This is where physical therapy comes in.

Now that their cast or brace has been removed, they need a therapist's help to strengthen their muscles so they can walk again. In fact, they may be out of their cast or brace, but still using crutches or a walker. For many people, this is a very slow and intentional process. They may see their therapist a couple times a week. Because they have not used the muscles in their leg for several months, they will start slowly, moving their leg in small ways and not putting much weight on their leg. Over time, they will increase the amount of movement, gaining strength through repetitive exercise. Little by little, they will become stronger and no longer need crutches. Then one day, their leg will be healed and they will walk as though they never experienced an injury.

When it comes to healing from betrayal, the process may look similar. Following discovery or disclosure, which dramatically fractures and injures the relationship, many partners will experience a period where they feel unprotected and unsafe. If they choose to join a group or get into counseling, it becomes the cast or brace that holds them in one place, so they are not vulnerable to further injury. And while they may feel immobilized in their relationship, this is helping them become more emotionally aware and stable. When the time comes to begin working on the relationship, this can feel like removing their cast or brace and getting into physical therapy. Although this may be a very slow process, it is the next step in the process that will help to strengthen the relationship, much like physical therapy helps to strengthen the muscles in an injured leg.

✚ How has your healing journey felt like a two-steps-forward-one-step-back process? Explain.

✚ In what way does this physical therapy analogy make sense with what you've experienced in this healing process?

_____
_____
_____
_____
_____

✚ What thoughts and feelings do you have about this journey being a slow process?

_____
_____
_____
_____
_____
_____

Healing from betrayal can be an excruciating experience that leaves many partners feeling overwhelmed and weary. Not only is it a process that takes time, but there seems to be an ebb and flow to the journey itself.

For partners who have chosen to stay in the relationship, they are continually navigating their own healing, as well as keeping up with the progress of their husband's recovery. It can be emotionally and mentally taxing when one day things seem to be moving forward at a great pace, but then relapse happens. And while this doesn't put the couple back to the starting line, it definitely can cause a pause in the progression. They will need to step back and take the time needed to process this specific issue before moving forward again.

The same can be true for partners who have chosen to leave the relationship or whose spouse has left the relationship. They can be moving along at a great pace and making strides in their healing, but then feel triggered by an anniversary date or a memory that pops up out of nowhere. They may need to pause and spend some time processing this specific issue with their counselor, group members, or safe friends.

✚ In any way, have you experienced a situation that caused you to pause
and process a specific issue? Explain.

_____

_____

_____

_____

✚ When this pause took place, did you seek any help from an outside source:
a counselor, pastor, group member, or safe friend? Explain.

_____

_____

_____

_____

_____

✚ If so, how did they help you restart your healing journey?
What tools and/or advice did they give you? Explain.

_____

_____

_____

_____

_____

On this healing journey, we are not alone. In addition to the support of the women in
this group, our heavenly Father has promised to help us. When we are weary, He will
help to carry our burdens and see us through.

Then Jesus said, "Come to me, all of you who are weary and carry heavy burdens, and I will give you rest. Take my yoke upon you. Let me teach you, because I am humble and gentle at heart, and you will find rest for your souls. For my yoke is easy to bear, and the burden I give you is light."

MATTHEW 11:28-30 (NLT)

✚ **How does this Scripture give you hope and encouragement for your healing journey? Explain.**

_____

_____

_____

_____

_____

As partners, it is important to remember that we are only responsible for our healing. We are only responsible for our choices and decisions in this process. We are not responsible for our husband's recovery, nor for the choices and decisions he makes in this process.

However, if we have children, they have likely been witness to the tension and/or impacted by what's happened in our relationship.

Scripture is clear about the consequences of a person's unhealthy behaviors and the way they contribute to unhealthy patterns within the family system. This is often the case when someone struggles with compulsive sexual behaviors.

You must not bow down to them or worship them, for I, the Lord your God, am a jealous God who will not tolerate your affection for any other gods. I lay the sins of the parents upon their children; the entire family is affected—even children in the third and fourth generations of those who reject me. But I lavish unfailing love for a thousand generations on those who love me and obey my commands.

DEUTERONOMY 5:9-10 (NLT)

This is why it's so important for those who struggle to work diligently on recovery to break this type of generational patterns and pursue a life of health and wholeness. It is a powerful truth that will allow parents to pass on good and healthy behaviors to their children.

For couples who choose to work on their relationship, they are off to a great start when a betrayed partner experiences healing and the addict establishes sobriety. However, healing the entire family will need to take place, if you want to experience the blessings Deuteronomy 5 speaks of:

> *But I lavish unfailing love for a thousand generations on those who love me and obey my commands.*
>
> DEUTERONOMY 5:10 (NLT)

At some point, this means disclosure will need to take place with your children too. If you have children living in the home, to some extent, they can feel the tension in the home, even if they don't know what's creating it. This is also true for partners who have chosen to leave the relationship or whose spouse has left the relationship.

Consulting with a trained counselor is essential before disclosing to your children. Disclosing to children is all about timing: making sure both parents have achieved an appropriate level of healing and recovery. Disclosing to children could go badly if the struggling spouse is still in denial or blaming his partner.

What Kids Need to Know

Disclosing to your kids should be done in an age-appropriate way, without giving specific details, but explained in a way they can understand.[23]

Preschool (ages 3-5): These children may have heard their parents fighting but don't know what's happening. They will need answers and reassurance around these types of questions:

- Are you going to leave me? Are you going to die?
- Am I in trouble?
- Do you love me?

This is also a good age to start the conversation about healthy sexuality. *How to Talk with Your Kids About Sex* is an excellent resource written by Rodney and Traci Wright and published by Pure Desire Ministries.

Early Elementary (ages 5-6): They will need answers and reassurance around these types of questions:

- Is this my fault?
- Will something bad happen? (Divorce?)

---

[23] Deborah Corley and Jennifer Schneider, *Disclosing Secrets: When, to Whom, & How Much to Reveal* (Wickenburg: Gentle Path Press, 2002), 141-142.

- Who are you now? (You are now very different and this child has learned to adapt to deprivation.)

Upper Elementary/Middle School (ages 9-13): They will need answers and reassurance around these types of questions:

- Am I normal? (They're thinking: How will this impact me?)
- Will I get this addiction because I have sexual feelings? (Another opportunity to reinforce what healthy sexuality looks like.)
- Will I become an addict because you are?
- If you get divorced, what will happen to me?

For Teens and Young Adults: They will need answers around these types of questions:

- How could you do this to Mom? To our family?
- How does this relate to me? ("You ruined my life.")

If you have older, adult children, there may be benefits to disclosing to them, especially if it means you are being obedient to the Lord and changing the potential generational curses into generational blessings!

✚ **What thoughts and feelings do you have about age appropriate disclosure for your children?**

✚ **How will this disclosure process bring about generational blessing to you and your family?**

Note: If you are feeling triggered by any of the lesson content or this healing process, and want to pursue professional help, please contact Pure Desire at 503-489-0230 or visit **puredesire.org/counseling**; or contact APSATS (The Association of Partners of Sex Addicts Trauma Specialists) at 513-874-2342 or email **info@apsats.org**.

7

What If He Doesn't Choose Recovery or If I Can't Move Forward ?

Healing in Motion

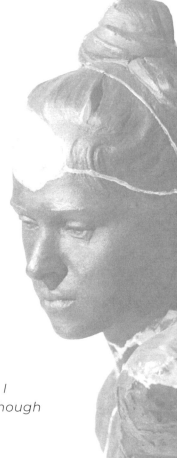

We pastor a large church and my husband is addicted to Internet porn. I recently found evidence on the computer that he is still looking at it although he promised he wouldn't. I can tell when he has been on the computer for several hours doing this; and then he will lie to me and say he is not struggling. He is a child of an alcoholic, which he had kept a secret from me for many years. We have been to counseling but when I brought up the Internet porn, he was furious with me. I have threatened that if he started doing this again, I would leave him. It seems he has lost any fear of consequences. I am not sure what to do. Should I kick him out, go tell the elders, divorce him, or just ignore this like I don't know it is happening?

CAROL

✚ From what you have learned about the healing process and healthy boundaries, what kind of advice would you give Carol? Explain.

Hopefully, after reading Carol's story you realize that she doesn't have a Safety Action Plan in place. While she is not responsible for her husband's recovery, her idle threats will not motivate him to change. In reality, he has experienced no consequences and probably doesn't believe she will leave, in spite of her threats.

As part of my advice to her, I said that he would not get better on his own. He is living a double life and God cannot honor it. If he continues without confrontation and real consequences, he will destroy himself, his family, and the church family. I then shared about how to put together a Safety Action Plan (which you learned about in Chapter 4, Lesson 3).

As a partner, one of the most difficult things you will need to do is follow through with what you have written in your Safety Action Plan. Otherwise you too may fall into the trap of idle threats. God has given us a divine plan that can help move the addict out of his addiction toward recovery. This plan is called the law of sowing and reaping.

In the early years of our marriage, I found myself interrupting this plan many times. I would pray for something to change and then a difficult consequence would come that could actually get Ted's attention and begin to cause change. But since I didn't like the consequences, I put on my Super-Wife mask and rescued us from fateful consequences. Many years ago, God began to deal with me about this. He said, *"Diane, I just answered your prayer with this difficulty. You rescued the situation and tied my hands from working in Ted's life."*

When I teach women about the Safety Action Plan and logical consequences, I talk about the law of gravity. I ask, "What will happen if I drop a book?" Of course, it will hit the ground. But, if we rescue, we catch the book in mid-air and keep it from hitting the ground. I confess, this is what I have done, interrupting the law of gravity and the law of sowing and reaping. I finally made a decision to stop rescuing and allowed difficult consequences to impact our finances. This became the turning point for Ted becoming very financially responsible. In fact, he has surpassed me in this area and is a fabulous steward of our finances. (I know this doesn't always happen and there may need to be different consequences, such as separate checking accounts.)

✚ **Share a time where you interrupted the law of sowing and reaping.**

_____

_____

_____

_____

_____

_____

_____

✝ Share a time where you allowed the law of sowing and reaping to take place and didn't rescue your husband and/or the situation.

_____

_____

_____

_____

_____

_____

_____

_____

_____

Two incidents of pastors and their wives come to mind when I think of the law of sowing and reaping.

The first couple moved to our city to go through the Pure Desire program. Part of the logical consequence (among other things) was that the pastor would not be in ministry for a year. At the end of the year, we would reevaluate those requirements depending on the severity of his addictive behaviors and his recovery progress. Six months into the recovery process, the husband wanted to play an instrument on stage during the worship services. His reasoning was that it wasn't preaching, so it should be okay.

Rather than reminding him of the guidelines, we asked his wife how she felt about it. Immediately, her frustration came to the surface and she said, "I am angry that he refuses to lead us in worship at home. All our family members play musical instruments and love worshiping, but he has not initiated any family worship for years. And now, he is insistent about being on stage. No, I don't want him to do this. It reminds me too much of the double life he has been leading as a pastor. I want to see him spiritually leading us as a family before he is released to any kind of public ministry."

I was so proud of this woman for sharing her honest feelings. This was a turning point for her husband as he began to realize that much of his self-esteem came from being "up front," getting accolades from other people instead of seeking God's favor and being a servant leader in his home first. Over time, he began to see that he not only used his sexual addiction but also his public life as a pastor to medicate his pain, rather than facing the issues that were driving his behaviors.

When the pain on the outside (natural consequences) becomes greater than the pain on the inside (trauma from the past), addicts are usually moved to change.

✚ Since discovery or disclosure, think about a time this statement has proved to be true. Explain.

_____

_____

_____

_____

✚ Has there been a time where you saw your husband make a change due to the external pain of a situation? Explain.

_____

_____

_____

_____

_____

The second couple also came to our church for recovery and healing. But within less than a month, the husband was upset because his children did not like being in a large Sunday school class. (They had come from a smaller church.) He came into the counseling session with a proposal to go to another smaller church where he would submit to their leadership, and thus his children would not have to experience so much pain.

I looked at his wife to see her response. I could tell she was caught between allowing her husband to create his own recovery plan and the consequences of seeing her children suffer. Talk about a Double Bind. I pointed out some observations:

- His acting out had not really stopped; he had cruised our red-light district the first week they had moved to our city but he denied that it was "acting out."

- Addicts love being in charge of orchestrating their own recovery process. It's part of their desire to control their life and avoid pain and consequences.

- Part of the logical consequences (the pain on the outside) would be to have him deal with the fallout of what was happening to his children. I suggested that he should go with them to class and help them integrate into a larger church.

Unfortunately, this wife gave in to his proposal and they went elsewhere for their recovery and healing. Within six months, he was involved in ministry at that church and within a year he was back in the pulpit of a new church. Two years later, their marriage ended and he was out of the pastorate.

✝ **With regards to the law of sowing and reaping (allowing consequences to do their job), why do you think this story ended the way it did? What could have changed the outcome?**

_____

_____

_____

_____

_____

_____

_____

Let me emphasize this truth: **Rescuing a person from the consequences enables them to continue in irresponsible behavior.** If your husband is not suffering the consequences, someone else is—usually you and your children. This truth is especially hard to consider when many women rely more on their husband for finances, home repairs, parenting issues, and more. When your husband doesn't help or provide, things get left undone, unpaid, unmended, and unresolved. In these cases, you may need to seek out specific help from wise counsel regarding what kinds of consequences would be appropriate. For example, if he has not repaired the washing machine as promised and you have to wash laundry by hand or at the laundromat, you are suffering. Consider what options might serve as appropriate consequences to get the repair taken care of: you might pay for the repair out of another fund. For those with more complicated circumstances, as mentioned, you may need to get sound counsel and consider consequences that work best for you, your needs, and your sense of safety.

God has called us to risk, not rescue. He has asked us to trust Him regardless of what those consequences yield. I think Queen Esther is one of the greatest examples in the Bible of a woman who was willing to trust God, regardless of the consequences.

When faced with the possible destruction of the Jewish people, she had to make the decision of confronting her husband, the King, with the truth. He had already eliminated one queen who dishonored him and if she confronted him with the truth, it could mean death for her. Her cousin, Mordecai, made this statement, "_Yet who_ _knows whether you have come to the kingdom for such a time as this?"_ (Esther 4:14). After much prayer and fasting on her part and the part of her people, Esther came to this conclusion, _"If I perish, I perish!"_ (Esther 4:16).

God did not cause the crisis Esther faced, yet because she was willing to risk regardless of the consequences to her own life, she and the Jewish nation were saved. Esther trusted God to intervene on her behalf and chose to do the hard thing.

✚ **Read the short book of Esther and explain your thoughts.**

_____

_____

_____

_____

_____

✚ **Explain the Double Bind she faced:**

_____

_____

_____

_____

✚ **Describe her wisdom in approaching her husband:**

_____

_____

_____

_____

_____

✚ **How was God faithful to Esther and her people?**

God has not caused the crisis you are facing. But like Esther, could He be challenging you to risk in spite of consequences, so that He can intervene?

✚ **What are you willing to risk to trust God to intervene on your behalf?**

Think about the situations you are facing and list the hardest things you have difficulty trusting God with the outcome. These should be actions and/or consequences where you have intervened and your husband didn't experience the consequences. Use the following chart to work through a Double Bind exercise, which will help you weigh the risk and determine potential outcomes to the situation.

Issue	If I intervene...	But If I let the consequences come...	Impact on him...	Impact on me...
Example: He stays up late playing video games and looking at porn, then has trouble waking up and getting to work on time.	*If I continue to intervene, I will feel stressed every time he doesn't go to bed at the same time, I will be afraid to be away from the house overnight, and he will continue his same patterns.*	*I risk the possibility of him becoming more addicted to porn and gaming. He could lose his job, which would create an extreme financial loss for us. We could lose our house and a lot more.*	*It is more likely he will grow and make new choices if he has the opportunity to face the consequences of his own actions.*	*I might still feel anxious (short term)... and will let go of holding all the responsibility.*

✚ What thoughts and feelings (fears) do you have about trusting God in one or all of the areas you listed?

_____

_____

_____

_____

_____

✚ If you choose to do the hard thing, what is one step you could take that would help you follow through with the consequences?

_____

_____

_____

_____

_____

✚ Write out a prayer asking for God's courage and wisdom, as Esther did in her time of crisis.

_____

_____

_____

_____

To some extent, healing from betrayal can feel like a matter of life or death. This is especially true if your spouse doesn't pursue his own recovery or if you can't move forward in your healing. Many partners are faced with this dilemma. But, if you are willing to identify and walk out the plan you create through the Three Circles, you will not only survive this season of life, but learn to live out the healthy life God has planned for you. The Three Circles exercise can help you determine activities that proactively contribute to your healing and help you to keep moving forward on your journey, regardless of the choices your spouse makes.

THREE CIRCLES[1]

The **Three Circles** exercise is designed to give you a very clear and convenient method of displaying all you have discovered so far about yourself and what you need to make strides in your healing. The explanation of the circles is followed by the actual graphic of the circles. You will write your own information in the circles based on what you learn from the explanation and examples.

The **INNER CIRCLE** describes experiences, coping strategies, and situations that cause you the most harm, fear, and lack of safety. **This is the area you're trying to avoid.** This includes thoughts, feelings, and behaviors you choose to avoid because they are harmful to you. The things listed in the INNER CIRCLE can become a fiery dart or weapon the enemy can use against you.

Inside the **INNER CIRCLE** write down the thoughts, feelings, and behaviors you want to avoid. This is a one-day-at-a-time process, where God is asking you to trust Him and walk TODAY by His grace. This is called the "manna" principle. When God led Israel out of Egypt, He supplied them with what they needed one day at a time. God will provide the grace you need one day at a time, but you have to know where to apply it, thus the priority of the INNER CIRCLE.

Your **INNER CIRCLE** might include:

- Looking through my husband's phone and/or email.
- Controlling/rescuing people or situations out of fear.
- Using anger and sarcasm to avoid addressing my true concerns and voicing my needs.
- Medicating my feelings of loneliness or worthlessness with food, alcohol, or drugs.
- Crossing my own boundaries to please someone else.
- Spending time in unhealthy places with unhealthy people.

---

[1] Sex Addicts Anonymous, *Three Circles*, 1991. While this tool was originally created for recovery, over the past 30 years, it has been used in many counseling arenas to help people find healing.

- Allowing myself to indulge in "dark thinking" and feelings of hopelessness.
- Avoiding connection and relationship with healthy women.

Next is the **MIDDLE CIRCLE**. These are the things that could potentially trigger you, leading you back to your INNER CIRCLE behaviors, which are harmful to you. The MIDDLE CIRCLE includes the thoughts, feelings, and behaviors that fall in the middle: between what is harmful to you and what is contributing to your healing and reflects the life God wants for you.

These **MIDDLE CIRCLE** behaviors can lead you back to the INNER CIRCLE, so developing strong boundaries and being intentional about living in health is imperative. In this circle, list thoughts, feelings, people, places, situations, and behaviors that you want to avoid because they trigger you.

Your **MIDDLE CIRCLE** might include:
- Feeling angry, isolated, or frustrated for an extended period of time.
- Allowing myself to spend time fantasizing about a better life.
- Overdoing all of it: overeating, overspending, overserving, over...
- Allowing black and white (all or nothing) thinking to dominate my thoughts.
- Pleasing others to feel good about myself.
- Being ticked off and cursing
- Procrastinating on daily/routine tasks.
- Allowing perfectionism to dominate my thoughts and behaviors
- Unable to say "no" and set healthy boundaries.

Finally, the **OUTER CIRCLE** is all about healthy behaviors that reinforce your healing. Write thoughts, feelings, behaviors, people, places, and activities that support your healing and the healthy boundaries you have in place. This might also include long term self-care behaviors and plans to maintain connection with others, especially after this Betrayal & Beyond group is finished.

Your **OUTER CIRCLE** might include:
- Regularly recite my specific personal promises God has given me.
- Read/listen to books on healing from betrayal, healthy boundaries, and other related topics.
- Spend more time having fun, whatever that looks like: alone, with my spouse, with my kids, and with friends.
- Learn to listen to myself and respect myself enough to set healthy boundaries.
- Explore new hobbies and interests in my life.
- Continue to expand my emotional awareness, identifying and expressing my feelings in a healthy way.

- Develop relationships with Christian women I admire.
- Develop healthy peer friendships with women who also desire a Christ-centered life.
- Develop a meaningful and deep devotional life.
- Focus on doing something healthy every day, not having an "all or nothing" mindset.
- Develop healthy eating habits and a workout schedule.
- Regularly spend time on self-care.
- Learn how to really relax when needed: spend time being still and silent.
- Use the FASTER Scale to become more self-aware and do a Double Bind when I find myself facing a challenge.
- Review my Three Circles weekly and stay in community with at least two women.
- Review my Safety Action Plan every few months and update it accordingly.
- Commit to going through Betrayal & Beyond again, possibly as a co-leader.
- Pay it forward to help others and eventually become a Betrayal & Beyond leader.

Here is an example of the Three Circles exercise:[2]

- **Inner Circle** - Behaviors and activities I want to avoid because they are harmful to me.
- **Middle Circle** - Behaviors or activities to avoid because they can lead me back to my Inner Circle.
- **Outer Circle** - Behaviors and activities that are healthy and support my healing.

---

[2] The Three Circles exercise used here is an adaptation of the Three Circles used by Sex Addicts Anonymous. The original is available through Sex Addicts Anonymous and pamphlets available online through the SAS store or by telephone or postal mail from the ISO office. www.sexaa.org.

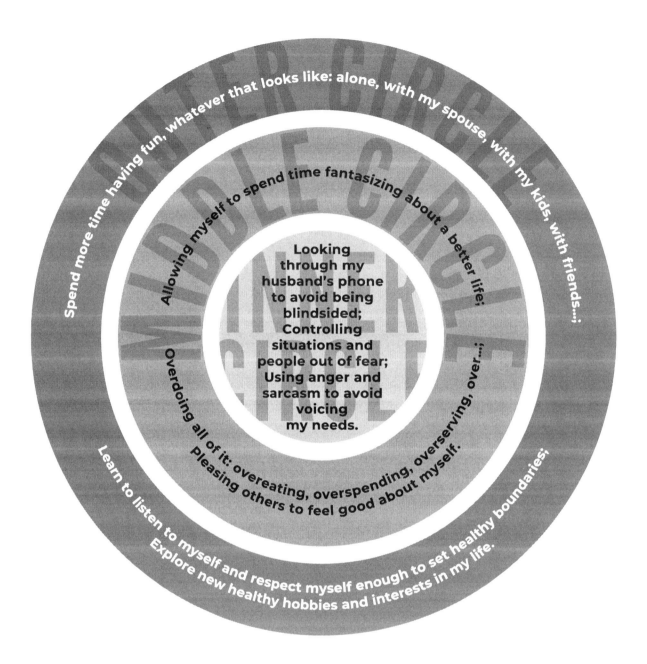

OUTER CIRCLE

Spend more time having fun, whatever that looks like: alone, with my spouse, with my kids, with friends...;

Learn to listen to myself and respect myself enough to set healthy boundaries; Explore new healthy hobbies and interests in my life.

MIDDLE CIRCLE

Allowing myself to spend time fantasizing about a better life;

Overdoing all of it: overeating, overspending, overserving, over...; Pleasing others to feel good about myself.

INNER CIRCLE

Looking through my husband's phone to avoid being blindsided; Controlling situations and people out of fear; Using anger and sarcasm to avoid voicing my needs.

✛ Now complete the Three Circles exercise using the next diagram provided.

Remember, this is a document in progress. At least once every three to six months you should revisit this exercise and adjust your responses to align with your current level of healing. You will find that this is an excellent indicator of the progress you have made and an invaluable tool in recognizing the progress you've made in your healing.

My Three Circles Exercise[3]

- **Inner Circle** - Behaviors and activities I want to avoid because they are harmful to me.

- **Middle Circle** - Behaviors or activities to avoid because they can lead me back to my Inner Circle.

- **Outer Circle** - Healthy behaviors and activities that are healthy and support my healing.

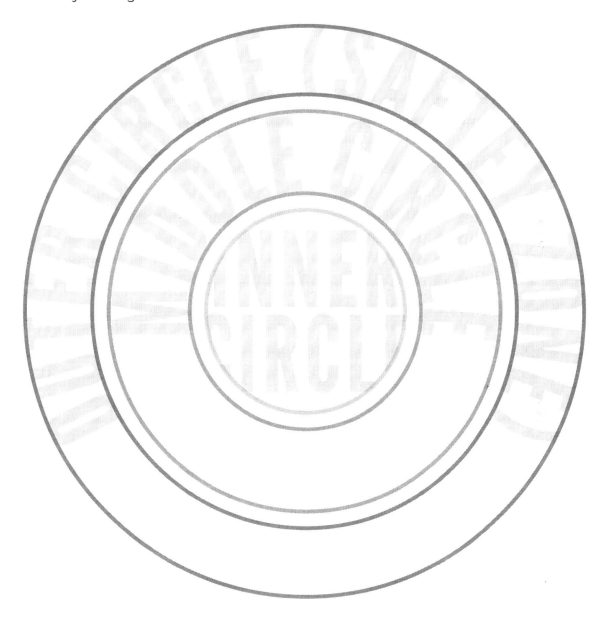

---

[3] The Three Circles exercise used here is an adaptation of the Three Circles used by Sex Addicts Anonymous. The original is available through Sex Addicts Anonymous and pamphlets available online through the SAS store or by telephone or postal mail from the ISO office. www.sexaa.org.

The Stages of Grief

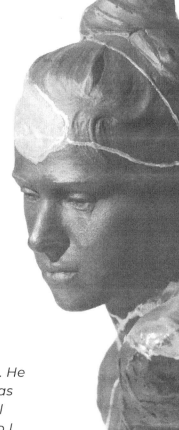

The husband I thought I had was a loving, hard-working, giving leader. He had integrity, was respectful, loved God...and loved me. Now I know I was living in a false reality. The real man is selfish, disrespectful, has no real relationship with God, and can lie as easily as breathe. The relationship I thought I had would stand the test of time and grow richer through the years. I was looking forward to growing old together in our home where we would enjoy our sons, their wives, and our grandchildren. Now, I don't know if I can even make it through today. The pain his actions have caused this family are horrific. He doesn't even see the damage he's done and, instead, acts as though everyone should go on and pretend nothing ever happened. The unity and fun are gone from our lives.

I used to love to cook, laugh, play games, sing, and have fun. I don't have the energy to do anything. What I force myself to do every day now feels so unreal—as though I am watching myself go through life pretending there is life, when all I really want is to no longer exist. His betrayal has killed my heart and yet somehow I still have to live. I know there are worse things others are facing and I shake myself and tell myself I am whining over nothing, get over it.

How can I even begin to grieve the loss of something I only imagined I had? How can I ever trust my own sense of reality? How can I trust God?

SARA

✚ What do you most relate to from Sara's story ?

Sara has so beautifully described the loss and doubt that a partner experiences when her heart and world have been crushed by the realities of betrayal. She has lost so much: what she thought was true about her husband, the life she thought they created, and even the future she thought they would have together. She's lost her joy and passion for life, her dreams of family and a future, her hope and ability to trust.

✚ What are some losses you've experienced because of the betrayal ?

I'VE LOST...

- ☐ My joy
- ☐ My sense of humor
- ☐ The ability to trust my own inner voice
- ☐ My best friend
- ☐ My innocence
- ☐ The way life was
- ☐ My ability to trust others
- ☐ Dreams of ministering with my husband
- ☐ Knowing what it would be like to be loved the way God wants
- ☐ My family's provider
- ☐ My home
- ☐ The ability to look at family photos without pain
- ☐ A godly example for my kids
- ☐ Self-confidence
- ☐ My ability to be around other women, especially pretty women
- ☐ My faith in people
- ☐ Financial security
- ☐ My future
- ☐ Other: _____
- ☐ Other: _____
- ☐ Other: _____

As Sara wrote in her letter, she began to look at her reality. She is pulling up the anchor that has held her captive. As she drags her anchor out of the murky waters of betrayal, she is unsure where to anchor her hope. Before she could tell herself, "I know there are worse things others are facing: I shake myself and tell myself I am whining over nothing...get over it." The denial she has expressed tells us that Sara is going through the stages of grief.

✚ **As you begin facing the reality of all you have lost, what are you afraid to look at? Explain.**

_____

_____

_____

Grief comes in stages. It comes in waves, rocking the boat we are on. It sometimes causes us to feel like we are caught in a hurricane; other times, like we are stranded on a desert island with our boat shattered in pieces too tiny to repair. Grief is not a smooth channel we can sail, with each stage following one right after the next. It is more like a roller coaster with unexpected twists and turns that thrust you in and out of stages, often with no forewarning.[4]

Stages of Grief[5]

Shock/Denial
Numbness, blanking out, avoiding thinking about "it."

Anger
Blaming someone or something, feeling injustice and rage.

Bargaining
Thinking "If I'd only..." and dealing with guilt, vain regrets of the past, and fear of the future.

Depression
Feeling hopeless, helpless, disappointed, isolated, and lonely. Inability to enjoy anything.

Acceptance
Embracing reality, forgiving and moving forward, forming new friendships while trusting God.

[4] Elisabeth Kubler-Ross was the first counselor to consider the cycles of dealing with grief. Her premier book On Death And Dying published in 1969 was groundbreaking regarding patients' needs and processes through difficult times. Her later works emphasized the "roller coaster" process of moving in and out of the stages, often visiting at least two if not all stages.

[5] Michael Dye and Patricia Fancher, _The Genesis Process: A Relapse Prevention Workbook for Addictive/Compulsive Behaviors_ (Auburn: Michael Dye, 1998), 115.

STAGE 1: SHOCK AND DENIAL

At first, it may be difficult for you to accept how you feel about being betrayed by your husband. Like Sara, you may tell yourself, "This isn't that bad. Others have it so much worse." In this first stage of grief you are stunned by the truth of what you have learned. You do not deny the event, but might deny how you feel about the event.

Here are three important truths regarding feelings and emotions.

01. My emotions reflect how I feel and are valid.

02. My emotions and feelings are not necessarily telling me the truth.

03. My feelings are not sin.

In this stage of grief, you may find yourself going into survival mode. You might try to stay so busy you don't have time to think about the betrayal and also become so exhausted you can hardly cope with life's daily tasks. You may withdraw from friends, family, and things you previously enjoyed. You may deny the realities of his hidden sexual behaviors and his betrayal, and how it is impacting you. You might find yourself saying something like, "Well, I struggle with my weight and my eating, so how can I blame him for his addiction?" However, this denial will gradually diminish as you look at the reality of all you have gone through and as you learn to express your feelings about the betrayal with other safe women and friends.

✚ **These words describe feelings you may have experienced while in shock and denial. Please check the words that are true for you now.**

☐ Surprised　　　　☐ Humiliated　　　　☐ Hurt

☐ Stunned　　　　　☐ Surviving　　　　 ☐ Frozen

☐ Shocked　　　　　☐ Lost　　　　　　　☐ Misunderstood

☐ Alarmed　　　　　☐ Restless　　　　　☐ _____

✚ **Choose one feeling you checked as true for you now and describe how it affects you or is present in your life.**

_____

_____

_____

_____

In John 16:20-33, Jesus prepares His disciples, closest friends, and companions for what they will soon experience as He goes to the cross to die for us all. He tells them they will weep and mourn and that they **will grieve**. Grief is painful. Jesus is preparing them for the experience. He compares the pain of childbirth to the grief they are about to endure. He assures them that, just like with childbirth, the end result of the pain is joy. He tells them:

> *I have said these things to you, that in me you may have peace. In the world you will have tribulation. But take heart; I have overcome the world.*
>
> JOHN 16:33 (ESV)

Grief has to be experienced and felt. It is painful. But if we are willing to go through all the stages of grief, we will come through it with a deeper level of joy that no one can take away (John 16:22). The outcome is healing for the heart and soul.

STAGE 2: ANGER AND FEAR

During this stage the most common question asked changes from "How could this have happened to me?" to "Why me?" You may feel angry at the injustice of the betrayal; you may project and displace your anger onto others. You may be experiencing new levels of fear and doubt. This is often accompanied by thoughts like: *What if he doesn't want to get healthy? What if he loses his job? What if he finds someone else and leaves me?* When given support, respect, and an opportunity to learn healthy ways of expressing your anger, fear, and the many other emotions that are present during this stage, you will eventually be able to move into the next stage of grieving.

✚ These words/phrases describe feelings you may have experienced during the anger and fear stage. Check the words/phrases that are true for you now.

☐ Scared	☐ Powerless	☐ Indignant
☐ Panicked	☐ Crazy	☐ Shamed
☐ Worried	☐ Out of Control	☐ Stupid
☐ Afraid	☐ Furious	☐ Devalued
☐ Sarcastic	☐ Mad	☐ _____

✚ **Choose one feeling you checked as true for you now and describe how it affects you or is present in your life.**

_____

_____

_____

_____

_____

At this point in your journey, one of the hardest things to do is to honestly look at your pain and losses and, at the same time, hold in perspective the truth that God has a future and a hope for you. The story of Admiral Stockdale brings home this point.[6] He was the highest ranking officer in the Vietnam POW camps. In his eight years of captivity and torture, he is credited with keeping many American service men alive so they could return home. When asked how he survived, he said, "You can never lose sight of where you want to be and believe you will ultimately get there. But while holding onto that belief, you can never stop looking at the fact of how bad things really are each day." He goes on to say that those who just looked at the future—"I'll be home for Christmas…, I'll be home for Easter…"—eventually, when that didn't happen, gave up and died. The others who only looked at the daily pain without the hope of future freedom, did not survive either.

This Stockdale Paradox is where you will find yourself. Every day will challenge you to look at the reality of your husband's hidden sexual behaviors and how it has impacted you—how it has cost you financially, relationally, emotionally, personally, and spiritually—while **at the same time** holding onto the hope that God is in charge and can make all things new.

✚ **Describe how this paradox applies to you personally.**

_____

_____

_____

_____

_____

[6] James Bond Stockdale, _Thoughts of a Philosophical Fighter Pilot_ (Stanford: Hoover Institution Press, 1995).

STAGE 3: BARGAINING

Many partners try to bargain with God. You may try to make deals and/or offer to give up an enjoyable part of your life in exchange for the return of your former relationship or the way life used to be. Or you may find yourself making bargains with the person who betrayed you: "I will do anything for you if you will only..." These efforts are vain attempts to restore life as you thought it was before the pain flooded in with reality, ugliness, and betrayal. It's common to bargain, even if futile, because our human nature wants relief from the pain.

✚ These words/phrases describe the bargaining stage of grief. Check the words/phrases that are true for you now.

☐ Pleading ☐ Bargaining ☐ If only...

☐ Begging ☐ Deal-making ☐ Terror

☐ I promise ☐ _____ ☐ _____

✚ Choose one word/phrase you checked as true for you now and describe how it affects you or is present in your life.

_____

_____

_____

_____

_____

_____

_____

STAGE 4: SADNESS AND/OR DEPRESSION

At first, you may experience a sense of great loss. Mood fluctuations and feelings of isolation and withdrawal may follow. It takes time for you to navigate what you're going through: gradually returning to your old self and becoming socially involved with what is going on around you. It's very difficult for partners to realize their "normal" is gone; and a new level of accepting and embracing your current reality must occur. In essence, as you go through this healing process, you're creating a new normal.

✚ These words describe feelings you may have experienced while in the sadness and/or depression stage. Check the words that are true for you now.

- ☐ Sorrow
- ☐ Depressed
- ☐ Tearful
- ☐ Helpless

- ☐ Abandoned
- ☐ Hopeless
- ☐ Sad
- ☐ _____

- ☐ Disengaged
- ☐ Empty
- ☐ Isolated
- ☐ _____

✚ Choose one feeling you checked as true for you now and describe how it affects you or is present in your life.

_____

_____

_____

_____

_____

_____

_____

_____

STAGE 5: ACCEPTANCE

Acceptance does not mean happiness. It is a willingness to believe that something is true (with no more denial) and it includes coming to terms with how it has changed your life (embracing the sadness). You accept and deal with the realities of the situation. This leads to hope. You are making decisions based on the present and the future, not on the past (before the betrayal). Remembering will be less painful and you can begin to look ahead to the future with a hopeful heart. You are deciding what your future will look like.

This is part of what Jesus meant when He promised that "your joy will be complete" (John 16:24). The word joy used here comes from the Greek root chairo, which means "to rejoice, be glad, to be well, to thrive." He intends for us to come through this and find wholeness and joy on the other side. This gives us great hope knowing His plans for us are good.

✚ These words are synonyms for "joy." Check the words you have experienced in your life. Then, circle one or two words you want to focus on as future aspects of joy in your life.

- ☐ Alleviation
- ☐ Cheer
- ☐ Ecstasy
- ☐ Festivity
- ☐ Gladness
- ☐ Jubilance
- ☐ Pride and Joy
- ☐ Regalement
- ☐ Sport
- ☐ Amusement
- ☐ Comfort

- ☐ Elation
- ☐ Frolic
- ☐ Glee
- ☐ Liveliness
- ☐ Prize
- ☐ Rejoicing
- ☐ Transport
- ☐ Animation
- ☐ Delectation
- ☐ Exultation
- ☐ Fruition

- ☐ Good Humor
- ☐ Luxury
- ☐ Rapture
- ☐ Revelry
- ☐ Treasure
- ☐ Bliss
- ☐ Delight
- ☐ Exulting
- ☐ Gaiety
- ☐ Indulgence
- ☐ Merriment

- ☐ Ravishment
- ☐ Satisfaction
- ☐ Treat
- ☐ Charm
- ☐ Diversion
- ☐ Felicity
- ☐ Gem
- ☐ Mirth
- ☐ Refreshment
- ☐ Solace
- ☐ Wonder

✚ Beginning this week, what can you do to cultivate joy in yourself and in your life?

_____

_____

_____

The stages of grief are not one-time events: "Whew, I made it through the sadness stage and now I'm done with that." You will find yourself cycling in and out of these stages sometimes in a matter of minutes. You might stay stuck in one stage for days, weeks, or even months depending on your specific situation. Each member of your family may experience these stages in their own way, at their own pace.

✚ If you have children, have you noticed any indication that they may be going through these stages of grief? If so, explain.

_____

_____

_____

_____

My Emotional Health and Healing

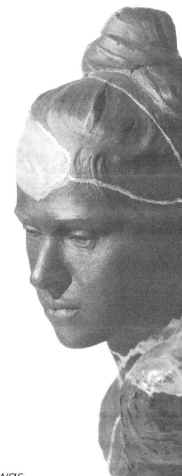

One night my husband didn't come home when he said he would; he was hours late. I laid on the couch, worried that he had been in an accident.

Late that night, I heard a noise at the door and jumped up to open it. He was heading out of the gate; I rushed out to him and he told me he was leaving us. He was crying and I begged him to come inside, terror rushing through my veins, I told him we could work it out, anything, but please don't leave me. He came inside and finally confessed he had gone to a prostitute, again. He told me how sorry he was, how devastated, how he hated his job, how he wanted to go to college. I was so scared, scared that he would abandon me and our three sons. I told him I would be willing to do anything for him and that I didn't want to lose him. I told him I forgave him and took him back into my heart and body that very night.

I shoved my feelings, pain, and fears into a closet in my mind and shoved the door closed. It was my job to love him unconditionally, and to assure him of my love, acceptance, and forgiveness. I couldn't have needs or feelings. I just had to try to be a better wife, to be more supportive of him, to do more for him, and then maybe he would not leave me.

Within two weeks we left our home and our extended family and moved to California where we didn't know a soul, so he could pursue his dream of going to college. I was relieved because there weren't houses of prostitution where we were moving and we were going to a Bible college, so surely "it" would never happen again.

It did happen again, coming in various forms—prostitutes, strippers, masturbation with porn calls, magazines, and Internet. The first time that he went to a "massage parlor" after our move was the first time that I truly understood this was an addiction.

I was angry, not outwardly, most of the time. I turned it inward, but my body was showing it as I lived with tremendous joint pain and exhaustion. I had gained so much weight; food was a comfort, an attempt to cover the pain that was hidden inside.

SHELBY

As Shelby's testimony indicates, when a husband initially discloses his hidden sexual behaviors, a partner's brain immediately propels her into survival mode: she is compelled to do and say whatever it takes to experience the least amount of pain in the moment. As a result, stress, fear, and tension can build up and may even cause physical illness.

While partner's experience a vast array of emotions during the initial stages following discovery or disclosure, anger tends to be a common response to betrayal.

By definition, anger is an emotional state that varies in intensity from mild irritation to intense fury and rage. Anger can be caused by external events, such as hurt created from a relationship or when we experience unmet expectations. Anger resulting from internal events can be more difficult to isolate because it is based on our own internal belief system, reactions to situations, our inner voice, and value systems. Anger is also a physical response that activates our adrenaline levels and hormones in our body, which is why many times it results in physical ailments.[7]

✚ **Take some time to evaluate your reactions and responses to situations that may result in anger. Is each statement true or false for you? Circle your answers.**

Anger Test[8]

T F **01.** I concern myself with others' opinions of me more than I would like to admit.

T F **02.** It is not unusual for me to have a restless feeling on the inside.

T F **03.** I have had relationships with others that could be described as stormy or unstable.

T F **04.** It seems like I end up helping others more than they help me.

---

[7] George Fink, *Stress: Concepts, Cognition, Emotion, and Behavior, Volume 1.* (London Wall: Academic Press, 2016), 289.

[8] Wanda Fisher, "Anger Test" (Eugene: Faith Center). Used with permission of Wanda Fisher.

T   F   **05.** I sometimes wonder how much my friends or family members accept me.

T   F   **06.** At times, I seem to have an unusual amount of guilt even though it seems unnecessary.

T   F   **07.** At times, I prefer to get away rather than being around people.

T   F   **08.** I realize I don't like to admit to myself how angry I feel.

T   F   **09.** Sometimes I use humor to avoid facing my feelings or to keep others from knowing how I really feel.

T   F   **10.** I have a problem with thinking too many critical thoughts.

T   F   **11.** Sometimes I can use criticism in a biting way.

T   F   **12.** I have known moments of great tension and stress.

T   F   **13.** Sometimes when I feel angry, I find myself doing things I know are wrong.

T   F   **14.** I like having times when no one knows what I am doing.

T   F   **15.** I usually don't tell people when I feel hurt.

T   F   **16.** At times, I wish I had more friends.

T   F   **17.** I find myself having many body aches and pains.

T   F   **18.** I had trouble in the past relating to members of the opposite sex.

T   F   **19.** Criticism bothers me a great deal.

T   F   **20.** I desire acceptance from others but fear rejection.

T   F   **21.** I worry a lot about my relationships with others.

T   F   **22.** I believe I am somewhat socially withdrawn.

T   F   **23.** I believe I am overly sensitive to rejection.

T   F   **24.** I find myself preoccupied with my personal goals for success.

T   F   **25.** I have often felt inferior to others.

T   F   **26.** Often I say "yes" and am upset at myself for not saying "no."

T   F   **27.** Even though I don't like it, there are times when I wear a mask in social settings.

T   F   **28.** I don't seem to have the emotional support I would like from my family and friends.

T   F   **29.** I would like to tell people exactly what I think.

T   F   **30.** My concentration sometimes seems poor.

T   F   **31.** I have had sleep patterns that do not seem normal.

T   F   **32.** I worry about financial matters.

T   F   **33.** There are times I feel inadequate in the way I handle personal relationships.

T   F   **34.** My conscience bothers me about things I have done in the past.

T   F   **35.** Sometimes it seems my religious life is more of a burden than a help.

T   F   **36.** There are times that I would like to run away from home.

T   F   **37.** I have had too many quarrels or disagreements with members of my family.

T   F   **38.** I have been disillusioned with love.

T   F   **39.** Sometimes I have difficulty controlling my weight, whether gaining or losing too much.

T   F   **40.** At times, I feel that life owes me more than it has given me.

T   F   **41.** I have a challenge controlling sexual fantasies.

T   F   **42.** To be honest, I prefer to find someone else to blame my problems on.

T   F   **43.** My greatest struggles are within myself.

T   F   **44.** Other people find more fault with me than they really should.

T   F   **45.** Many of the nice things I do are done out of a sense of obligation.

T   F   **46.** Many mornings I wake up not feeling refreshed.

T   F   **47.** I find myself saying things that I shouldn't have said.

T   F   **48.** It is not unusual for me to forget someone's name after I have just met them.

T   F   **49.** It is difficult for me to motivate myself to do things that don't need to be done.

T   F   **50.** My decisions are often governed by my feelings.

T   F   **51.** When something irritates me I find it hard to calm down quickly.

T   F   **52.** I would rather stay at home and isolate than be with other women socially.

T   F   **53.** I would rather watch a good sporting event than spend a quiet evening at home.

T   F   **54.** I am hesitant for people to give me suggestions even though they are good.

T   F   **55.** I tend to speak out whether someone wants to know my opinions or not.

T   F   **56.** I would rather entertain guests in my own home than be entertained by them.

T   F   **57.** When people are being unreasonable, I tend to take a strong dislike to them.

T   F   **58.** I am a fairly strict person, liking things to be done in a particular way.

T   F   **59.** I consider myself to be possessive in my personal relationships.

T   F   **60.** Sometimes I could be described as moody.

GUIDE TO THE ANGER TEST

How many of the 60 statements did you mark True? _____

What your score indicates (your total number of statements marked **True**) about you and anger:

1-15	Extremely healed or in denial
15-30	Normal range
30-40	Needs or circumstances are pressing
40+	Needs help through counseling for trauma or specific issues

It is not unusual for women going through a *Betrayal & Beyond* group to score 30 and above, depending upon the level of trauma they have experienced through their betrayal. Other areas of hurt and trauma of the past that haven't been processed can also cause a higher score.

The numbers below reflect statements that deal with **boundary issues**. They indicate times when you might be overreacting or underreacting to situation.

4   6   7   11   13   15   18   26   29   33   33   38   45   47   50   56   58

How many of the 16 boundary statements did you mark True? _____

The numbers below reflect statements that deal with **self-esteem issues**. Unresolved hurts from the past can create insecure responses in the present.

1   5   19   20   21   22   23   24   25   27   43   53   54

How many of the 13 self-esteem statements did you mark True? _____

✚ After taking the Anger Test and reviewing your results, what thoughts and feelings are you experiencing?

_____

_____

_____

_____

_____

✚ We all learn to express anger in one of two ways. Circle the response that best describes your anger and determine whether your anger is more repressed (anger turned inward) or explosive (anger turned outward).[9]

While this is not an exhaustive list, it may give you an indication of how you typically respond when feeling anger.

Repressed Anger	Explosive Anger
Very easily hurt	Critical and cutting
Afraid to say "no"	Never listen to others viewpoints
Think everything is my fault	Must be the best
Feel used; "doormat" mentality	Demand my own rights
Usually a loner, a form of hiding	Argumentative
Easily depressed	Lack compassion
Don't know how to have fun	Self-centered and judgmental
Usually fearful	Hold grudges

[9] Wanda Fisher, "Repressed or Explosive Anger" (Eugene: Faith Center). Used with permission of Wanda Fisher.

Repressed anger turns inward, causing depression, low self-worth, and low self-esteem. While this may be a response intended to protect us, it often ends up causing extreme internal pain. Explosive anger turns outward, attacks others, and often ends up hurting relationships. Neither response is healthy, yet both are normal responses to pain and trauma.

Emotions are part of us. Each time we suppress our emotions they become like bricks on a protective wall inside of us. We hide behind the wall to protect ourselves from harm. Anger is often one of the least safely expressed feelings, and therefore is frequently repressed.

✚ **Which category of anger (Repressed Anger or Explosive Anger) do you most identify with? Explain.**

_____

_____

_____

_____

_____

_____

Contrary to many teachings in Christian circles, **anger is not bad**. It is an emotion God gave us as a gift—a natural inner warning sign to alert us to greater issues. Just like a stop sign on a roadway, anger causes us to stop and look around for dangers. Anger alerts us to nearby emotional hazards. If we heed our own anger stop signs and look within, we will often find the underlying feelings that need to be addressed. Doing so allows us to stay healthy in our heart, mind, and spirit. Anger is a very healthy stage of grief and can indicate we are starting to acknowledge the losses that have occurred, thus validating the pain and healing process.

As you continue reading Shelby's story, consider her process of working through anger.

I asked Jesus to help me remember everything I needed to process. The door to the bulging closet full of my feelings, pain, fear, anger, and grief burst and all of the contents fell to the floor around me. Journaling those stored up feelings enabled me to express what I had tried so hard to keep inside. Some of my words were written with so much anger that the paper tore underneath my pen. I taped in painful notes my husband had written to me during our separation and divorce, writing how I felt about them on the same page.

Through it all, Jesus never left my side, giving me the freedom to "get it all out." My last page was a prayer: "Please remove the revenge in me, Lord. There is so much pain in me and in my heart; I can see it in my sarcasm. Oh Lord, please soften my heart with Your oil, open my eyes to see, fill me with understanding, soften my heart to receive. I want all that You have for me, Jesus."

And He showed me that every page of my notebook was a car on the freight train that had frightened me. Each hurt I released was like a car that dropped off the back of the train. Car after car fell off until all that was left at the bottom of the hill was the engine—the last page, my prayer. And I could stop the engine, step down from the train, and freely walk away, hand in hand with Jesus—Who would never leave me or forsake me.

SHELBY

✚ **What pictures come to mind when you think about your experience with anger? Draw them here.**

+ Explain your drawing.

_____

_____

_____

_____

_____

_____

_____

We all experience anger in one form or another and need to learn how to express our anger in a healthy way. This happens by becoming more emotionally aware, being able to identify and name our feelings in the moment. It also happens when we are able to communicate our feelings in a way that fosters relationship.

Most people don't like conflict and work very hard to avoid any type of confrontation. But through this process of healing from betrayal we've learned that our feelings matter and we have a voice to express our feelings in a healthy way. **A better way to think of confrontation is engagement.** When we use confrontation in a healthy way, we are intentionally engaging in the relationship to bring about a solution. We are moving toward the other person, moving toward a continued relationship with them.

As you consider this list of Strategies for Confrontation, think of this in the context of engagement; intentionally engaging to build relationship.

Strategies for Confrontation

EXPLAIN YOUR PERCEPTIONS:

- Be very specific.
- Say exactly what happened, when, where, and how often.
- Don't describe your emotional response at this point.
- Don't generalize or use abstract or vague terms.
- Avoid accusing the other person of bad intentions or motives.
- Other: _____

EXPRESS YOUR EMOTIONS:

- Speak calmly and at a normal volume.
- Use "I" statements that center on your emotions, perceptions, and thoughts.
- Say how you feel about the situation, not about the person.
- Don't go to extremes in processing (e.g. denial or unleashing rage).
- Avoid putting the other person down or using shame.
- Don't attack the entire character of the person.
- Other: _____

SHARE THE NEEDED CHANGES:

- Ask for something the person can actually do.
- Request only one or two small, practical changes at a time.
- Be specific about the behaviors you want to see stopped and those you want to see continued.
- Don't merely imply that you would like a change.
- Don't ask for too big a change or too many changes at a time.
- Consider the other person's needs.
- Avoid assuming only the other person has to change.
- Other: _____

EXPLAIN WHY:

- Say exactly how their change in behavior will help you.
- Explain how implementing the change will benefit them, too.
- Give appropriate boundaries and consequences if their behavior doesn't change.
- Don't be ashamed to say why you want the change or why it's important to you.
- Avoid threatening or bullying.
- Other: _____

✚ **Name three of the strategies for confrontation you can already do.**

01. _____

02. _____

03. _____

✚ **Name three of the strategies for confrontation with which you struggle, typically leading to unsuccessful confrontations.**

01. _____

02. _____

03. _____

When there cannot be an appropriate demonstration for the anger and confrontation with the person, it will be important for you to find a healthy way to release the anger. **Studies on women and anger have shown that those who cannot complete the release of anger-related energy compound it within themselves causing tremendous damage to their bodies and minds.** All of the following are common in women who continually repress anger: tumors, depression, skin disorders, as well as gastrointestinal, circulatory, and respiratory illnesses.[10]

When anger is extremely high, it's critical to be creative in releasing the anxiety and pressure. Consider these options:

- Engage in strenuous work or exercise, according to your physical capability.
- Write and write and write (and cry) to get all the feelings and frustrations out (like Shelby did).
- Vent with a safe friend. Allow her the opportunity to give you some feedback about themes, assumptions, and internal conflicts she might hear in your tirade; it could prove tremendously helpful to you.
- Seek professional counseling to work through anger and betrayal trauma.
- Do a deep breathing exercise. Breath deeply in and out for 5 minutes without moving your chest. Only your stomach should move—deep diaphragmatic breathing.
- Rehearse your personal promises: words God spoke to you personally (through experiences with God) with Scripture that matches your personal word.
- Use art to express your anger.

The important thing is to give yourself healthy, balanced outlets to express anger so you don't internalize it or become violent.

---

[10] Judith Worell, *Encyclopedia of Women and Gender: Sex Similarities and Differences and the Impact of Society on Gender* (San Diego: Academic Press, 2002), 143-146.

✚ What proactive strategies have you learned in this lesson for processing anger?

_____

_____

_____

_____

_____

_____

_____

_____

_____

_____

_____

_____

_____

_____

_____

_____

_____

_____

_____

Note: If you are feeling triggered by any of the lesson content or this healing process, and want to pursue professional help, please contact Pure Desire at 503-489-0230 or visit **puredesire.org/counseling**.

8

CHAPTER EIGHT

What is Forgiveness and Reconciliation ?

When Will I Be Able to Trust Again ?

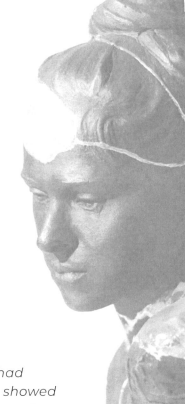

What is Forgiveness ?

I met and married a wonderful guy who showed me Jesus in a way I had never experienced before. I fell in love with him and with the Jesus he showed me. He shared his heart, his frustrations and temptations, his dreams and desires, his pain and pleasures. We were best friends and from the beginning of our marriage served in ministry together. As a new believer I took Jesus' words in Matthew 6 very seriously when it talks about the connection between me not forgiving others and God not forgiving me. I knew I sinned daily in my thoughts, words, impatience, anger, and selfishness.

A few months after our second son was born my husband called me while he was away on a work trip and confessed that he had just gone to a prostitute. He was so repentant, so broken, crying, he told me he was so sorry. I wanted to be a "good Christian" wife. And, after all, God forgave me every time I asked; didn't I have to forgive him when he asked? I was afraid if I didn't forgive him, that God would not forgive me. So, still in shock, still on the phone, I told him that I forgave him, but that if he ever cheated on me again I would leave him.

I remember lying on the couch all night sobbing and shaking but I thought, "Well, he finally sowed his wild oats, found out how empty it was, and promised he would never do it again." Yet I felt so defiled. Questions slammed into my heart and mind. Why did he do this? Why would he pay someone for what I gave him so freely, so lovingly, so passionately? There were no answers to the haunting echoes of doubt that entered my heart and soul.

SHELBY

So what is forgiveness? Is it mandatory? Is it a giant eraser that is supposed to help us forget what has been done to us? What does it mean to forgive and forget, anyway? Is it a one-time event? Is it possible to forgive too soon?

✚ **What phrases, thoughts, and feelings run through your mind when you think about what it means to forgive?**

_____

_____

_____

_____

_____

_____

_____

_____

_____

Before we define forgiveness, let's look at common myths about forgiveness.

Forgiving does NOT mean...

Myth One: I approve of what was done.

As we learned in previous lessons interfering with the consequences of another person or enabling their unhealthy behavior is often due to a lack of healthy boundaries. In John 8, Jesus meets a woman caught in adultery. He forgives her for her sin, but then He tells her to leave her life of sin. He did not approve of her choices and clearly communicated this to her and forgave her.

Myth Two: I excuse, minimize, or justify what was done.

When Moses led the people toward the Promised Land, he was constantly dealing with their complaining, blaming, and rebellious choices. God told Moses, "_I will strike them down with a plague and destroy them, but I will make you into a nation greater and stronger than they._" Moses could have eliminated the problem and was offered a great future. But Moses appealed to God on their behalf and God forgave them. Moses did not justify their behavior, make excuses for it, or make the wrong they were doing look right. (See Numbers 14.)

✚ Write about a time when you made excuses, minimized, or justified something done to you, like Shelby did when she thought her husband had "finally sowed his wild oats."

_____

_____

_____

_____

_____

_____

_____

_____

_____

Myth Three: I "turn a blind eye" to what was done or deny it altogether.

Teri: 1 Corinthians 13:5 says that love "keeps no record of wrongs." For years, I felt guilty every time I read this verse because I longed to love my husband like this. However, the intense pain of his betrayal would still be there. I worked hard to deny the betrayals and turn a blind eye to this reality. I told myself, "*Well, he is such a good person in these other areas, so this latest 'little indiscretion' is not that bad. It could be so much worse.*"

Forgiving someone who has wronged us may require that we bring to light their inappropriate or sinful behaviors. The Greek word for "wrongs" in this verse is *kakos*, which means evil. It is the same word Jesus used in Mark 7 when He tells us what makes us "unclean." Since it is evil, we must acknowledge it rather than denying it or pretending it didn't happen.

Myth Four: I "forget" and pretend I'm not hurt.

A few years later my husband confessed that he had gone to a prostitute a second time, but this time he hadn't told me on the day he did it. He'd done it a year before, during a time when things were not going well in our marriage. Now I didn't know what to do: I had told him that I would leave him if he ever did that again. So, I went to our pastor for counsel and he gave me this advice: since it happened in the past and my husband apologized, saying he would never do it again, I should forgive and forget and never bring it up again. Then I would be forgiving like Jesus. So I vowed to be just like Jesus, I would forgive and forget.

SHELBY

After Moses asks God to forgive the people (Numbers 14), God replies, "*I have forgiven them as you asked. Nevertheless...*" and God goes on to explain the consequences that would still occur because of their sin. So even God did not "forgive and forget." They were forgiven, yet they would still suffer the consequences for their sins. It's an example of a spiritual law that governs our world: the law of sowing and reaping. It is God's way of teaching us cause and effect in relationships.

When Jesus taught us how to pray (Matthew 6), He never said, "...forgive men and forget when they sin against you..." It is impossible to forget meaningful events in our lives, regardless of whether they are negative or positive. God created our brain with a memory that permanently stores emotionally-laden events. **When betrayal happens to you, the memory of the discovery and/or disclosure will be stored in your brain along with your emotions and other details of the event. It becomes a part of who you are.**

Think of it this way: if you had a huge bleeding cut on your body, you wouldn't pretend it was not there. Betrayal carves huge, gaping wounds into your heart, mind, and life. Just like a large wound on your body, you must address how deep it is and determine what has invaded it to cause contamination. You must treat the wound, sometimes reopening it to clean out deep, hidden infections. You often need to ask for outside help to understand what is happening inside the wound and allow others to help you treat the damage done. Only with careful cleaning, dutiful tending, and consistent nurturing can such a wound begin to heal properly. The same is true when dealing with the trauma from betrayal.

✚ Think about a time when you told someone you forgave them, but later found yourself hurting over what had been done. Explain the situation. To which of these myths were you responding?

Myth Five: I must reconcile with the person who hurt or betrayed me.

Although the Bible clearly shows we *always* need to forgive, this is not the same as reconciliation. God forgave the whole world and yet the whole world is not reconciled to Him (John 3:16-21). When Jesus died on the cross for our sins, He made a way for us to be reconciled to God. He made it *possible* to reconcile, but first we have to make a choice to repent for the things we have done and the sins we have committed. This leads us to a key point about reconciliation and forgiveness:

To be reconciled with someone, there must be repentance from the wrongdoer. Reconciliation takes two people. Forgiving only takes one person.

When you make the choice to forgive someone, it is **vertical**—directly between your heart and the heart of God. On the other hand, reconciliation is **horizontal**; it occurs between you and another person, and *both* people must be active participants in the process. Therefore, reconciliation isn't always possible since it depends on the two addressing the issues honestly and coming back together to reestablish healthy boundaries and earn trust once more.

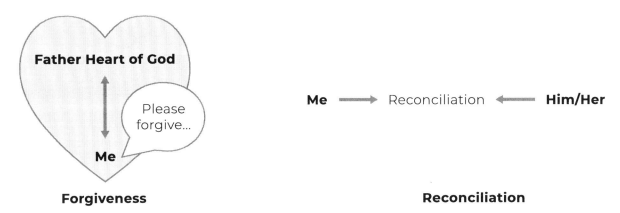

As you can see from the images, forgiveness and reconciliation are two different things. They are not even opposite sides of the same coin; they are different coins in the same monetary system.

Myth Six: I am pardoning the person who hurt or betrayed me.

To pardon means to release a person from liability for an offense. It is releasing them from punishment and/or from debts that are owed. A person is pardoned by someone who is in a high position of authority, like a governor or judge. **The person doing the pardoning is not a part of the offense, but holds an outside, objective view.**

Forgiveness happens between the two people who are directly involved in the offense. It begins vertically, when you ask God to give you a forgiving heart toward the person who has hurt you. God's forgiveness and grace then flow into your heart and spirit and THEN can flow horizontally to the offender. It may never bring about reconciliation with the offender, but inside you will be free to walk in forgiveness. **Ultimately, only God can pardon.**

✚ **Which of these six myths did you think defined forgiveness?**
How did this affect you?

_____

_____

_____

_____

_____

Now that we've explored several myths about forgiveness, let's consider some key truths to help illuminate the reality of forgiving.

Forgiving...

Truth One: is hard.

Jesus models what forgiveness looks like. Unlike us, He NEVER sinned. Yet He physically took on the consequences of our sinful choices when He died for you and me. (He _really_ understands what it is like to suffer because of others' bad choices!) He was willing to suffer and die for you and me, who did sin and would continue to sin! He died so that you and I could be forgiven. Going to the cross was excruciatingly hard and it cost Jesus everything. Forgiving is not easy; it is painful.

Forgiveness is ferocious love dripping with freshly spilled blood. Forgiveness is a heartbreaking choice to love the sinner more than you hate the sin.[1]

Truth Two: requires us to look at the truth.

To forgive someone who has betrayed you, you must look at what was done without any denial: you must look at the truth of how you have been wounded. As with any deep wound, you must take off the bandage and address what's in there. If left untreated, it can create an infection and illness in you, the wounded one. For those who have experienced betrayal, examples of "infection and illness" may include bitterness, low self-esteem, envy, self-hatred, resentment, revenge, sarcasm, depression, and hatred. When left untreated, these "infections" can spread like cancer, causing death to your spirit and mind, if not your body.

---

[1] Laurie Hall, _An Affair of the Mind_ (Wheaton: Tyndale House, 1996), 218.

During His last supper with His disciples, Jesus told them that one of them would betray Him. Judas, who had already made arrangements to betray Jesus, responded to Him, "*Surely not I, Rabbi?*" Jesus answered him, "*Yes, it is you.*" Jesus knows intimately what it feels like to be betrayed. Even to the point of being betrayed with a kiss. He told the disciples, "*This very night you will all fall away on account of me.*" Then, when Peter swore that he would never do such a thing, Jesus gave him very specific details of how Peter would abandon Him. *Jesus spoke truth* to all of them about how they would betray and abandon Him (Matthew 26).

Only Jesus knew the details of His betrayal before it happened. We must look back at how we were betrayed, address the truth of what was done, and identify how it has impacted our life. All of the layers of betrayal may not have been revealed yet, but we must look at the truth of what we know today.

Forgiving takes time; it is not instantly given. Jesus did not immediately tell his disciples that He forgave them. It was later, in the midst of His greatest suffering on the cross, that He cried out, "Father, forgive them..."

If you take care of yourself and walk with integrity, you may be confident that God will deal with those who sin against you. Above all, don't give birth to sin yourself; rather, pray for those who persecute you. God will one day turn your persecution into praise.[2]

Truth Three: is a choice, not a feeling.

Christ on the cross chose to forgive when He pleaded, "*Father, forgive them, for they do not know what they're doing*" (Luke 23:34). His body was racked with the pain of the physical beatings He had just endured. He had heard their accusations, hatred, and lies against Him. Yet, He saw beyond all of it to the truth that the very people who had made all of those terrible choices really did not understand the ramifications of their vicious, angry words and actions. We, too, can choose to forgive even when we are not pain-free.

Forgiving is a choice. Working through the grief cycle to acceptance will be more difficult if we're holding on to unforgiveness. We have to grieve and mourn our losses and work through our feelings of anger and pain to be set free, but it starts with a choice to forgive. Choosing to not forgive keeps us stuck in limbo: where we cannot have the past as we thought it was and we cannot yet embrace the future as it will be.

Forgiveness is the key to letting go of the past and being able to move on to a new future.

---

[2] Warren Wiersbe quote, *76 Quotes About Forgiveness*, https://www.christianquotes.info/quotes-by-topic/quotes-about-forgiveness/.

✚ **Think of a time when you knew you should forgive someone, but didn't feel like it. Explain your experience.**

_____
_____
_____
_____
_____
_____
_____
_____
_____
_____
_____
_____
_____
_____
_____
_____
_____
_____

Truth Four: starts with you and God.

Jesus took three disciples to support Him and pray with Him during His greatest time of need. Despite that, Jesus returned more than once only to find them asleep. They didn't really understand what He was going through. I believe He really wanted their support and that is the reason He kept waking them up. Yet He struggled alone, on His face, crying out to His Father in Heaven. Forgiving can be very lonely. This is often true for those who have experienced betrayal trauma.

No one completely understands the agonizing pain you are going through—not your best friend, not your family, and not the person who betrayed you. **When you forgive someone you are taking part in a miracle that hardly anyone will notice.** No one can record this miracle on Facebook or in a digital photo because it happens in the privacy of your inner self, silently, invisibly between your heart and the heart of Father God.

None of us are there yet, but if we each have this attitude, we will put to death our reactions to criticisms and offenses. And though we may still stumble, we will learn that carrying the cross is not merely dying to self; it is embracing the love of Christ that forgives the very ones who have crucified us, that the battle that comes against us has actually driven us into the embrace of God.[3]

Truth Five: is a process.

The decision to forgive is the beginning of a process. It is simply your agreement to examine what this whole betrayal has cost you. Like the layers of an onion, each layer of the betrayal will need to be looked at, grieved, and forgiven. As each layer slips away, it will allow a deeper layer to show.

Here is a powerful testimony from a person who chose to forgive:

The layers terrified me. How much more could there be? Would the layers never end? I felt the stench of the onion burning my eyes and the scent of it destroying my soul. Yet, one day, I realized the layers were a tender expression of God's incredible love for me. He knew that I could only handle one layer at a time, and having to deal with everything that had happened (the whole onion) all at once would destroy me. So He lovingly allowed me to see one layer at a time, when He knew I was ready to handle it. Now when He reveals another layer to me, I get excited, not about how painful and "stinky" it will be, but because I know it means He believes I am now ready and able to deal with it. Each layer has become proof that I have grown!

TERI

Peter came to Jesus and asked how many times he had to forgive when his brother sinned against him (Matthew 18:21-22). Jesus answered him, "*Seventy times seven.*" I believe Jesus was letting Peter know about the onion! Forgiveness is an ongoing process, piece-by-piece, layer-by-layer.

Often, with betrayal, you will find out more truths along the way. Most men who struggle with compulsive sexual behaviors do not disclose all the details at one time. They think they are somehow making the process less painful by telling their wives the whole truth in smaller bits and multiple disclosures. Although staggered disclosure can be more painful, the reality for us is that we may not know the whole truth about the betrayal, this side of Heaven; but we can choose to continue to move toward healing by not allowing unforgiveness to destroy our own mental and physical health. This allows God's Spirit to continually cleanse us, grow His fruit within us, and lead us in His truths so we can live in health.

---

[3] Duke Taber, *The Power to Forgive: 21 Christian Quotes on Forgiveness*, Francis Frangipane quote, https://viralbeliever.com/christian-quotes-on-forgiveness/.

✚ Describe a time when your choice to forgive happened through a more extended process. Consider your initial age at the time of the event and how more truths of the event were revealed over time. Describe your own growth and development since then and the continued actions of the offender(s).

_____
_____
_____
_____
_____
_____
_____

Truth Six: leads to freedom.

Forgiving allows you to be set free from the internal chaos that often accompanies unforgiveness. When you have worked through the process of forgiving, it allows you the freedom to be who God made you to be, open and transparent, and not stuck in the woundedness created by betrayal.

✚ Based on what you have learned in this lesson, what aspects of forgiveness are new for you? How does this give you hope and inspiration for your future?

_____
_____
_____
_____
_____
_____

Is Reconciliation Even Possible After Betrayal ?

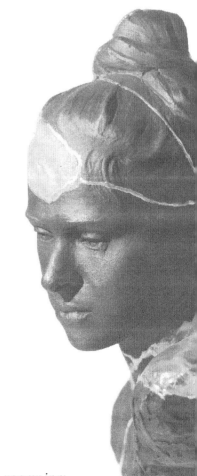

There was a time early in my Christian walk when I did not know the meaning or purpose of forgiveness. I truly thought it meant I had to forgive and forget. The pain that I had experienced for so many years living with my husband's addictions to pornography, drugs, and spending were far too much to forget. I thought I would have to reconcile with him if I forgave him and I could not bear not having him know just how badly he had hurt me. I felt I had been the victim of his choices and I placed the blame of my hurts on my husband.

When I joined this group, I began to understand that the purpose of forgiveness is to become aligned with God. God wanted me to understand that there was freedom from being a victim and that by forgiving I could be released from the bondage of being a victim. I began to forgive my husband and our healing began.

Two years into our relationship's restoration, my husband came home after his Seven Pillars of Freedom group and confessed to me that he had not told me everything; time stopped, I was afraid to even breathe. He said that confessing this would allow him to be completely free and that the Holy Spirit had been pressing him to release himself from his own bondage.

LIZ

✚ In what way(s) can you relate to Liz's story?

The process of forgiving is mysterious. Our unique path to forgiveness may look different for each of us. We may work to forgive someone who has hurt us and even get to a point where we think we're done with the process, only to be blindsided again by something that triggers a point of trauma still connected to the experience. This is often evident by the way we respond to a triggering situation. We may respond excessively or aggressively, or maybe become non responsive, either way responding in a way that is out of the ordinary or uncharacteristic for us. When this happens, it gives us more opportunity to dig deeper and heal another hidden layer of our trauma.

✚ Think of a recent time when your response to a situation was clearly a trauma response. Explain.

✚ **Why do you think you responded this way ?**

My husband then confessed that he had three affairs early in our marriage, one of the women being my best friend. He seemed so repentant and also very relieved to have the chains of this secret broken. I immediately broke down in tears and for the first time in my life experienced true depression. But the Lord had taught me the steps I needed to take to be free of the pain.

For the first couple of days, I found myself rolling in and out of the stages of grief. I looked carefully at the losses this new disclosure brought into my life and I allowed myself to grieve. I exposed my anguish to God and to my husband. I made the choice to forgive.

I wrote a letter to my best friend within days of my husband's disclosure. I prayed, asking God to help me find the right words. I told her about sexual addiction and shared with her about my complete faith in the Lord. I told her how much she had hurt me and then I explained that I was forgiving her for what she had done.

LIZ

In many ways, forgiveness allows us to move beyond living our life as a victim. When we have deep wounds, we need to face the wrong committed against us, choose to forgive, and work toward the day when the pain and trauma of the experience no longer has power over us. Whether our relationships survive or not, **this single decision to work toward forgiveness empowers us and builds inner resiliency.**

When we have experienced betrayal at the hands of the ones we love and trust, we feel victimized. Liz was a victim of betrayal by both her husband and her best friend. She had the right to blame the people who hurt her for bringing pain and destruction into her life. It was not because of anything she had done, yet she suffered painful consequences because of others' choices. Remember, when we choose to forgive, we are not condoning the wrong, nor does our forgiveness require us to have a relationship with someone who has been abusive or is an unsafe person.

Forgiveness is not a feeling - it's a decision we make because we want to do what's right before God. It's a quality decision that won't be easy and it may take time to get through the process, depending on the severity of the offense.[4]

When others have committed great offenses against us, it is difficult to come back, to rise up again, and face the world with confidence. We must decide if we will continue to live life as a victim or if we'll take charge of our lives.

As we learned in the previous lesson, forgiveness and reconciliation are two different things. Forgiveness first happens vertically: it's the process of realigning and restoring our relationship with God after we've experienced pain and hurt from another person. Reconciliation happens horizontally: when we choose to forgive the person who hurt us and we work *together* to bring our relationship back to health.

True reconciliation is never cheap, for it is based on forgiveness which is costly. Forgiveness in turn depends on repentance, which has to be based on an acknowledgment of what was done wrong, and therefore on disclosure of the truth. You cannot forgive what you do not know.[5]

When exploring this process of forgiveness and reconciliation, it's important to recognize that **reconciliation takes two people working together to reach a common goal**. Reconciliation will not happen if only one person is doing all the work to invest in the relationship, and the other person is not.

✚ **At this point in your relationship, how likely is reconciliation?**

1	2	3	4	5
Not Likely		Possible		Highly Likely

---

[4] Joyce Meyer, BrainyQuote, https://www.brainyquote.com/quotes/joyce_meyer_454432?src=t_forgiveness.

[5] Statement by Archbishop Desmond Tutu on his appointment to The Truth and Reconciliation Commission, November 30, 1995.

✚ Give some examples of why you chose this number/answer ?

_____

_____

_____

_____

_____

✚ If reconciliation is possible/highly likely, what things need to take place for this to happen in your relationship ? Explain.

_____

_____

_____

_____

_____

Choosing to forgive someone allows our heart to begin to heal. It rips off the scab of numbness on our heart and allows God to come and cleanse the "infection" in that wound. When we choose not to forgive someone, the scab remains and the infection continues to fester and grow, contaminating other parts of us. So choosing to forgive someone who has hurt us is beneficial to us.

While it may feel like there is a sense of control by not forgiving, we are unknowingly attached to the person who hurt us by chains of unforgiveness. Instead of walking forward freely, we drag these chains with us affecting every part of our life and interfering with our ability to make strides in our healing.

When we choose to forgive, it impacts our heart, soul, and mind. Research suggests that the act of forgiving is associated with positive emotional responses compared to unforgiveness.[6] Using fMRI, results indicate that giving forgiveness activated areas

---

[6] Ricciardi, Emiliano et al. "How the brain heals emotional wounds: the functional neuroanatomy of forgiveness." _Frontiers in human neuroscience_ vol. 7 839. 9 Dec. 2013, doi:10.3389/fnhum.2013.00839

in the brain involved with compassion, empathy, and emotional regulation, relieving associated feelings of anger and resentment.

When we choose to forgive, we begin to clearly see and acknowledge the evil that has been done. Forgiveness is a choice to release our right to sit in judgment of the offender and return that right to God.

> *Do not take revenge, my dear friends, but leave room for God's wrath, for it is written: "It is mine to avenge; I will repay," says the Lord.*
> ROMANS 12:19 (NIV)

✚ **How would forgiving free your spirit? Describe the spiritual battle within you over the issue of forgiveness.**

_____

_____

_____

_____

_____

_____

❝❝ *The person who gains the most from forgiveness is the person who does the forgiving.*[7]

In Luke 4:18, the Greek word *aphesis* means forgiveness. But in this particular verse it is translated as both deliverance and liberty. Isn't it interesting that deliverance and liberty are directly tied together with forgiveness?

> *The Spirit of the Lord is upon me, because he hath anointed me to preach the gospel to the poor; he hath sent me to heal the brokenhearted, to preach deliverance [aphesis] to the captives, and recovering of sight to the blind, to set at liberty [aphesis] them that are bruised.*
> LUKE 4:18 (KJV)

---

[7] Kendall, *Total Forgiveness*, XXXIII.

We have talked about the spiritual benefits of forgiveness, but what about the physical benefits? According to Dr. Michael Barry, a pastor and the author of the book, *The Forgiveness Project*, harboring unforgiveness changes our immune system.[8]

He once stated in an interview:

Harboring these negative emotions, this anger and hatred, creates a state of chronic anxiety. Chronic anxiety very predictably produces excess adrenaline and cortisol, which deplete the production of natural killer cells, which is your body's foot soldier in the fight against cancer.

Barry said the first step in learning to forgive is to realize how much we have been forgiven by God.

When a person forgives from the heart, which is the gold standard we see in Matthew 18, we find that they are able to find a sense of peacefulness. Quite often our patients refer to that as a feeling of lightness.

✚ Of the Scriptures in this lesson, which one was most impactful to you and why?

✚ If you could totally forgive, what would be the greatest benefit or blessing for you?

[8] Michael Barry, *The Forgiveness Project: The Startling Discovery of How to Overcome Cancer, Find Health, and Achieve Peace* (Grand Rapids: Kregel Publications, 2011) 80.

✚ Since discovery or disclosure, what experience has shown these benefits to be true?

_____
_____
_____
_____
_____
_____
_____
_____
_____

✚ From God's perspective, why do you think He wants us to have a forgiving heart?

_____
_____
_____
_____
_____
_____
_____
_____
_____
_____

Rebuilding Trust

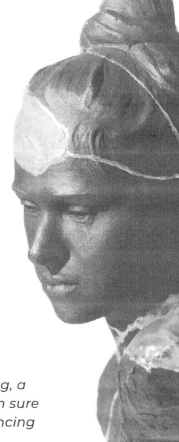

Learning about my husband's affair with my best friend was something, a few years ago, I would have told you I could not imagine surviving. I am sure it would have been the death of my marriage. Now, here I was experiencing the painful reality of one of my greatest fears. Sending the letter to my friend was a part of my grieving process, letting her know how much she had hurt me and telling her that I forgave her was important to my own personal healing. It took away the judgment and contempt I felt toward her and I believe it helped break the soul-ties[9] that both my husband and I had with her.

LIZ

Learning that your husband is having an affair can be one of the most painful things a woman can experience in this life. As Liz stated, it was something she believed she could not survive. She was betrayed not only by her husband but also by her best friend. His infidelities had broken her trust in him and now she was also afraid to trust other women, even very close friends. The ripple effect of betrayal impacts many people from the ones involved in the infidelity to their spouses, children, family, and friends.

We have learned that forgiveness is one of the steps on the path toward reconciliation. Not only for a partner and her spouse, but for others who may have been involved with the betrayal.

---

[9] Soul-ties refers to the physical, emotional, and spiritual connection formed between sexual partners. This will be discussed further in this lesson.

✚ In the following table, write in the names or initials of everyone you need to forgive—all who have been, in any way, involved in your betrayal. Then check the appropriate box to the right: are you ready to forgive or not yet?

Person	Ready to forgive	Not yet
	☐	☐
	☐	☐
	☐	☐
	☐	☐
	☐	☐
	☐	☐
	☐	☐

Some other people you might want to consider adding to your list are:

- Well-meaning people who gave wrong and sometimes hurtful advice.
- Those involved in pornography, both creating it and posing for it.
- Christians who judged or avoided you because of the betrayal or your spouse's addiction.
- All those who participated in the betrayal(s).
- Relatives who added to the pain by lecturing or giving their opinions about you or your marriage.

As you read, Liz wrote her best friend a letter expressing hurt over the affair between Liz's husband and her best friend. She also extended forgiveness to her friend. Liz received this response:

Dear Liz,

Needless to say, I was surprised to receive your letter, but felt the truth should come out in order for you and your husband to go forward in your relationship. I am truly sorry that I have hurt you. You deserve an apology and I do not deserve your forgiveness. I am so grateful for it, though.

I do know what it feels like when your husband cheats on you; it is devastating. But it must be so much worse knowing he did it with me, your best friend. I wish I could take it all back. I do not know of any way to make amends to you. If you need to call me and tell me what you really think of me that would be okay. Please do whatever you need to do to heal.

How you found it in your heart to forgive me, I will never know. You deserved much more from me. Although you have told me you forgive me, I know this is something that you will never be able to forget and that makes me very sad. Please let me know if there is anything I can do or say that would help you get through this.

Receiving this letter validated the pain and loss I had experienced. Hearing her admit how much she had hurt me, and how sorry she was, validated that she had been my friend. Reading her words was like a cleansing for me; I could now be at peace and rest. I was able to give closure to what had happened in the past. I was able to let the past become the past, at last.

I redeemed myself by choosing to forgive her; she redeemed herself by confessing the truth. The power the secret of their affair had held over us for fifteen years was finally and forever broken. The destruction of that secret, of which the letter was the culmination, was the beginning of the complete restoration of my marriage. Once the soul-tie with her was broken, I was able to begin to rebuild trust. It launched my husband and me from slow, small steps toward healing to rapid healing. My husband and I are now experiencing a deeper friendship and intimacy than I ever dreamed was possible.

LIZ

Liz and her husband no longer have any relationship with the friend. They chose to let go of the friendship, recognizing that it would be unsafe for their marriage and personal healing. They each made the choice to forgive, which led to the restoration and rebuilding of their marriage. Liz's husband risked the possibility of the destruction of their marriage and shattered the power of secret shame when he confessed the whole truth to Liz and asked her to forgive him. He also had to work to forgive himself for the act and the subsequent years of deceit. Liz, after allowing herself to fully grieve, shattered the power of the secret when she chose to forgive both her husband and her former best friend. Choosing forgiveness allowed them to move beyond guilt and blame, focusing all their energy on moving forward in their relationship together.

Forgiving someone should be very specific:

- I forgive him for lying to me and keeping his secret for so many years.
- I forgive him for using porn and masturbating.
- I forgive him for visiting a prostitute.
- I forgive him for giving me a venereal disease.
- I forgive him for breaking our wedding vows and having an affair.
- I forgive him for sexting and sharing pictures of his body with other women.

Forgiving each transgression validates the pain of each wrong and marks our ability to process and overcome the wrongs done to us. For this reason, **we cannot forgive transgressions we don't know about. We cannot fully forgive unless we know *everything* for which we need to forgive.** This is why forgiveness is a process: when full disclosure takes place and we have all the information we need to make informed decisions, we are better prepared and able to choose the path of forgiveness.

 Love doesn't erase our memories. It is actually a demonstration of greater grace when we are fully aware of what occurred— and we still choose to forgive.[10]

Obstacles to Forgiveness: Soul-Ties

Soul-ties are obstacles that can hinder your relationship and true intimacy. We encourage you and your spouse (if you have chosen to work toward reconciliation) to pray over past soul-ties that might still be hindering your relationship with each other.

In her testimony, Liz stated that forgiving her friend for having an affair with her husband became easier once her husband broke the soul-ties with Liz's friend. If infidelity has occurred, soul-ties must be broken.

When we have sexual intercourse, soul-ties are formed. Genesis 2:24 (KJV) says that we "become one flesh" and Matthew 19:3-10 (NIV) also says we are "no longer two, but one." This is a profound mystery (Ephesians 5:32) that goes beyond neurochemical bonding in the brain, physical familiarity, and emotional intimacy to a complex bonding that occurs in the spiritual realm.

In the Pure Desire Sexy Christians Seminars, I share a powerful illustration of soul-ties and how they impact us.[11] I take a pink and a blue piece of paper and glue the two together. When it is almost dry I pull the papers apart; in that tearing process,

---

[10] R.T. Kendall, *Total Forgiveness* (Lake Mary: Charisma House, 2002), 18.

[11] Ted Roberts and Diane Roberts, *Sexy Christian Seminar*, Pure Desire Ministries International, puredesire.org.

some of the blue is left on the pink paper and some of the pink is left on the blue paper. God intended our sexual relationship to literally glue us together as husband and wife. If infidelity has taken place, there are still attachments between the lovers due to the neural imprints of their sexual, emotional, and physical unions, as well as the thought patterns associated with their relationship. The enemy can use these attachments as hooks that continue to jerk the spouse around, even if they have removed themselves from the relationship. BUT God can heal and restore ANYTHING.

> *Do you not know that your bodies are members of Christ himself? Shall I then take the members of Christ and unite them with a prostitute? Never! Do you not know that he who unites himself with a prostitute is one with her in body? For it is said, "The two will become one flesh." But whoever is united with the Lord is one with him in spirit.*
>
> *Flee from sexual immorality. All other sins a person commits are outside the body, but whoever sins sexually, sins against their own body. Do you not know that your bodies are temples of the Holy Spirit, who is in you, whom you have received from God? You are not your own; you were bought at a price. Therefore honor God with your bodies.*
>
> 1 CORINTHIANS 6:15-20 (NIV)

As you can see from this Scripture, when a person engages in sex outside their marriage, the sin is not only against God and their partner, but also against their own body. For sexual freedom to resume between a couple, it is important that **the struggling spouse walk through these steps of praying** for the soul-ties to be broken:

- Ask forgiveness for sinning against God (Psalm 51:3-4).
- Ask forgiveness for sinning against their own body (1 Corinthians 6:18).
- Ask forgiveness for sinning against the affair partner's body (1 Corinthians 6:18).
- Ask forgiveness for sinning against their spouse's body (Matthew 5:23-24).

Remember, God wants to heal every area of our lives through this process. As we continue to give Him all our pain and woundedness, He will restore us to walk out His plan and purpose in our lives.

HOW CAN I EVER TRUST AGAIN?

It has taken incredible courage on your part to break through the wall of deception created by your husband's compulsive sexual behaviors and venture into a place of truth where you can again trust your instincts and the Holy Spirit to give you guidance on your healing journey.

Steps Toward Building Trust[12]

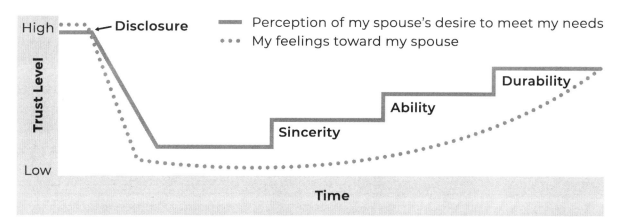

As you look at the Steps Toward Building Trust graph, notice that when you were first married not only were feelings for your spouse high, but also your hope that he could meet your emotional needs. When discovery or disclosure happens, it is normal to see the lines on the graph plummet, indicating that your love for your spouse has been nearly extinguished. Your hope for him to meet your needs has also bottomed out due to the painful reality of betrayal.

Usually when discovery or disclosure happens, the addict will begin to do anything to keep the marriage. Notice on the graph how he can begin to show sincerity and ability, and yet your feelings for him can still be nil. He could even walk on water and begin doing everything you have wanted him to do in the past and you still may have no feelings of love toward him. This is normal because your pain and trauma from the betrayal is so deep. Lastly, observe how over time he proves some durability through consistent behavior and new healthy habits, thus becoming more trustworthy. At this stage, most women can dare to trust his love once more.

From the chart you can see that for trust to begin to be established, you must see a **sincere** heart. A sincere heart expresses repentance and chooses to turn in a new direction. Because of his heart's callousness, he may not initially grieve the impact of his compulsive sexual behaviors, but instead desire to escape it and sense relief that he can stop pretending. Believe it or not, his "hidden life" has required enormous amounts of energy and vigilance. The addict is generally very relieved to give up this burden.

A sincere heart is not just turning in a new direction, but also is moving forward with energy. Notice how Scripture attaches actions as outward evidence of guarding your heart, mouth, eyes, and feet:

---

[12] DeLoss Friesen and Ruby Friesen, *Counseling and Marriage: Volume 19* (Dallas: Word Publishing, 1989), 36.

Keep vigilant watch over your heart; that's where life starts. Don't talk out of both sides of your mouth; avoid careless banter, white lies, and gossip. Keep your eyes straight ahead; ignore all sideshow distractions. Watch your step, and the road will stretch out smooth before you. Look neither right nor left; leave evil in the dust..

PROVERBS 4:23-27 (MSG)

One major action step for him would be his willingness to be accountable to a group of men, such as a Pure Desire recovery group, going through *Seven Pillars of Freedom*, and possibly seeking counseling.

✚ **What actions have you seen that would help you to trust his words? Or, if he hasn't started the recovery journey, what actions would you need to see to rebuild trust in his words?**

_____

_____

_____

_____

Additionally, you must see that he has the **ability** to follow through with what he has committed to do to begin rebuilding trust. You will need to see him acquiring new attitudes, behaviors, and skills to rebuild relationships that have been damaged. Ability does not just mean doing what is required in his men's group, but rather seeing evidence that he is beginning to grow and change emotionally and spiritually.

Expansion of his abilities could be evident in all areas of his development. Remember, most addicts stop growing emotionally at the point their addictions take over. They are no longer using their energy toward problem-solving, long-term thinking, discernment, and delaying gratification. However, when an addict stops using addictive methods to medicate their pain and starts choosing to pursue health, you will see small changes in different areas of their life at first. For example, you might notice he is listening more and processing the conversation more than he did before. You may notice he is talking more frequently and has more in depth conversations with men, which is a tremendous first step in learning to build friendships with other men instead of isolating. This growth requires energy, vulnerability, and learning new ways of dealing with almost every area in his life, and he is attempting to do this without medicating like before. Remember, he has probably been in an addicted state for years—possibly decades—and even small changes take incredible effort and show hope.

✚ What new skills have you noticed your husband working on in the following areas: his relationship with God, you, and others; vulnerability and honesty in discussions; his work around the house, job, career, and parenting; and other areas? If he is just beginning the recovery process, what new skills would you like to see him working on?

_____

_____

_____

_____

_____

_____

_____

_____

_____

_____

Finally, you will need to see **durability** in his commitment to wholeness, which will require him to not only learn, but master healthy habits. You have to know he's doing these things for himself and his relationship with God. Otherwise, it will feel like placation again: a key aspect of additive relationships. Only time will tell if he is really ready to embark on this lifelong journey of healing.

Realize that it will take awhile before in-depth oneness can be re-established in the relationship. As previously mentioned, Dr. Patrick Carnes has done research in studying sex addicts through their recovery process and has found it takes an average of three to five years for transformative healing to take place. However, many addicts experience significant behavioral changes within the first 60 days of recovery.

Our experience at Pure Desire Ministries places us in agreement with Dr. Carnes, recognizing that most men start compulsive sexual behaviors decades prior to disclosure or discovery. Real lasting change happens slowly but surely. The fog begins to lift as truth shines through. The pain begins to recede as new healthy relationships develop and accountability is embraced. **It is the addict's job to regain your trust over the next couple of years through a long-term commitment to health.**

✚ In what areas of your husband's life have you seen him commit
to a goal despite difficulties?

_____

_____

_____

_____

_____

_____

_____

✚ How might this give you hope for the future? If you are not currently
married, how might this information give you hope and a healthy perspective
about future relationships?

_____

_____

_____

_____

_____

_____

_____

_____

✚ What reactions, feelings, and perceptions do you have after learning about the "Steps Toward Building Trust" and its effect on your relationship?

_____

_____

_____

_____

_____

_____

_____

_____

_____

_____

_____

_____

_____

_____

_____

_____

_____

_____

_____

_____

_____

_____

Note: If you are feeling triggered by any of the lesson content or this healing process, and want to pursue professional help, please contact Pure Desire at 503-489-0230 or visit **puredesire.org/counseling**.

9

God's Promise of Redemption is for Me, Even if I Can't See it Now.

A Vision for the Future.

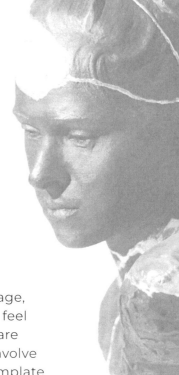

LESSON ONE

A Plan for My Future

Despite the work you are investing into healing yourself and your marriage, your husband may not be moving in the same direction. Many partners feel anger, anxiety, and fear as they consider and plan for their future. Here are two examples of letters I have received over the years. Both situations involve husbands who violated their marriage vows causing the wives to contemplate divorce. Read each letter carefully and decide what advice you would give them.

Dear Diane,

After discovering the affair five months ago, we talked a lot about how the marriage could come to this. I felt the Lord was leading me to forgive and love him. He was surprised I didn't kick him out and now thinking back, I don't remember him feeling truly remorseful. At that time, he promised he would never see her again. This week, I found out he visited her. He said he just wanted to tell her how well his business is going and how lucky he was to have a wife like me who would forgive him. He finally admitted she is a stripper and he paid for a lap dance. We have agreed to separate, but I'm not sure I can stay in this relationship. Should I divorce him?

STACY

✚ What are your thoughts about Stacy's decision ?

_____

_____

_____

_____

_____

_____

_____

_____

As you read through Trina's letter, think about how she approached her situation differently.

Dear Diane,

I have not believed in the validity of divorce for Christians, but don't know what else to do. We had been separated for a year because of his multiple affairs and got back together six months ago because he said he was willing to do whatever it takes. While we were apart, I was resolved to deal with my trauma and pain, regardless of his choices. I have gone through the Betrayal group twice and had the support of many wonderful women. I spent time working on developing healthy coping strategies, finding my voice, and, in the process, put into place healthy boundaries and a Safety Action Plan. I have grieved the loss of our once happy marriage and had hoped things would be different after a year of separation.

For him to come back, he had to agree to go to a Pure Desire men's group which he started doing before we got back together. He also needed to agree to monthly counseling and a polygraph. He said "yes" to everything and did all these things before we got back together. Just recently he has complained about not liking the accountability group at our church and has decided to go to another church and join a regular men's group that isn't focused on sexual issues. He has also made excuses for canceling two counseling appointments. He said he did what I asked him to do and I should be happy about that. I feel I have given him a chance to change and I have been using the new tools I gained through my healing process. The last straw came when he started drinking again (which was one of the areas he was accountable for in his Seven Pillars of Freedom group) and hanging out at bars, all hours of the night. Since this behavior led to previous affairs and he has violated my Safety Action Plan, I see no other recourse but divorce.

TRINA

✚ What are your thoughts about Trina's decision?

_____

_____

_____

_____

✚ Compare and contrast the choices made in the lives of these two women. Explain your reasoning.

_____

_____

_____

_____

_____

✚ What advice would you give to Stacy?

_____

_____

_____

_____

✚ What advice would you give to Trina?

_____

_____

_____

_____

The natural consequence of a separation by Stacy could possibly give her husband a wake-up call and move him out of denial. But she has no support system, no Safety Action Plan, and has not exhausted other possibilities including a men's group for him and/or counseling for the two of them.

Trina had a Safety Action Plan that she continually referred back to in the hope of restoring fidelity in their marriage. From her husband's response, it is obvious he wants the marriage on his terms and isn't serious about doing whatever it takes. Trina was also wise to give herself time to heal and slowly move toward reconciliation. Trina has grounds for divorce (as noted in Matthew 5:31-32 and 1 Corinthians 7:15, which state that infidelity and abandonment are reasons to consider divorce). These Scriptures imply that there are ongoing acts of infidelity. Domestic violence and ongoing abuse would also be grounds for divorce. Look back at Chapter 4, Lesson 2 for definitions of abuse in the Abuse Inventory. Although Trina has grounds for divorce, I would encourage her to meet with her pastor or counselor (one who understands sexual addiction) and continue to seek the support of women for spiritual guidance in the process of making her decision.

Look back at your Safety Action Plan (Chapter 4, Lesson 3). Check any of the following questions that you may need to spend more time thinking through.

- Does my plan include specifically how I will respond if there is a relapse?

- Is my plan realistic in light of how long an addict's healing process takes (e.g. three to five years)?

- Have I clearly stated what I need from my spouse in order to trust again?

- Have I clearly communicated steps I need to see him taking, and the natural consequences that will take place, if he is not proactive in the healing process?

- Have I sought God for His wisdom and direction even if I have biblical grounds for divorce?

- Have I sought the professional wisdom of a Christian counselor or pastor who understands sexual addiction? (Remember, your small group is there for support, encouragement, and to be a sounding board; however, they are not equipped to counsel you.)

- Is my support system adequate enough to allow me to follow through with whatever the natural consequences are?

- Do I have plans for continued support when this group ends?

✝ **What questions from this list, or others that have come to mind, do you need to process and add to your Safety Action Plan?**

_____

_____

_____

_____

_____

_____

_____

_____

_____

_____

Divorce should be the last resort. As we pursue godliness in our lives, doing the right thing is usually the hard thing.

Seeking the Lord's will and wise counsel will be advantageous, whether you choose to stay married or choose to divorce. As you are pondering the questions to which you just responded, the following Scripture and Laurie Hall's comment might help you fine-tune your Safety Action Plan:

> *Do not be wise in your own eyes; Fear the Lord and depart from evil. It will be health to your flesh, And strength to your bones.*
>
> PROVERBS 3:7-8 (NKJV)

Laurie states in her book, *Affair of the Mind*, that deciding what to do is like laser surgery; only things that directly affect you must be sliced off. In other words, if your spouse has been irresponsible in keeping you safe financially, you may need to take charge of things that directly affect you and the children (e.g., car insurance for your car, health insurance for you and the children).

...Perhaps you pay your own bills, file a separate tax return, or take your name off joint charge accounts if money isn't being handled wisely. This is not being controlling. This is being responsible for your own issues.[1]

---

[1] Laurie Hall, *Affair of the Mind* (Colorado Springs: Focus on the Family, 1996), 184.

✚ Since discovery or disclosure, what steps have you taken to create safety in your environment and safety as you continue to move forward in your healing?

_____

_____

_____

✚ What impact has this had (or will this have) on your plans for the future?

_____

_____

When we committed to this healing journey, we likely had no idea where we would be today. But God knew. As we listened to His Spirit prompting us and stepped when He said step, He has faithfully led the way, even during the most difficult times. We have trusted Him with our healing so far, and we can trust that He has the best plans for our future.

As you contemplate what your future holds, meditate on the following Scriptures. Answer the questions below.

> _Trust in the Lord with all your heart_
> _And do not lean on your own understanding._
> _In all your ways acknowledge Him,_
> _And He will make your paths straight._
>
> PROVERBS 3:5-6 (NASB)

✚ Based on where you're at in your healing journey, what are you trusting God for today?

_____

_____

For our present troubles are small and won't last very long. Yet they produce for us a glory that vastly outweighs them and will last forever! So we don't look at the troubles we can see now; rather, we fix our gaze on things that cannot be seen. For the things we see now will soon be gone, but the things we cannot see will last forever.

2 CORINTHIANS 4:17–18 (NLT)

✛ **As you continue to heal from betrayal, what things are you looking forward to in the future?**

And I am certain that God, who began the good work within you, will continue his work until it is finally finished on the day when Christ Jesus returns.

PHILIPPIANS 1:6 (NLT)

✛ **What areas in your life is God continuing to work on that make you excited and hopeful about the future?**

What If Your Marriage has Already Ended?

As I listened to their story, I could not even look up. My heart was pounding with so much pain that I thought it literally might burst. Tears poured down my face as I sat and silently suffered through the pain. These questions slammed my heart and mind: "Why wasn't I worth it? Why would these men choose their marriage, but the man I loved did not? And what is so bad about me that my husband did not want me, but instead walked away?"

If you are feeling that same kind of pain, I am so sorry...the freight train of sadness hurts so much! The "why" questions that had been trapped in my heart had also been binding me to a victim mentality. Those questions, trapped in my heart, had held me captive on the tracks of grief, unable to embrace the sadness and move on to acceptance. Stuck on those tracks, when I heard someone mention "marriage," or saw a husband put his arm around his wife or show affection, it felt like an arrow struck my heart. It was as if those trapped questions defined who I was.

Believing I was "not worth it" and "so bad" was keeping me from being able to walk forward into who I was to become. But now, I have experienced a deeper level of healing than I ever thought possible. Now, when I hear stories of restoration, I feel great joy for the marriages that have survived.

TERI

✚ **What thoughts and feelings do you have after reading Teri's story?**

_____

_____

_____

✚ **If your marriage has already ended, how can the women in your group be praying for you?**

_____

_____

_____

Moving Forward in Health

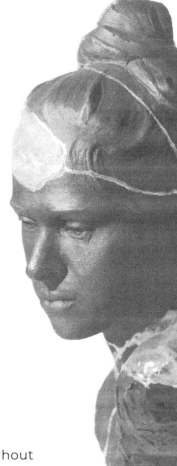

This poem, taken from *Behind the Mask*, was written by Jessica. Throughout the book, Jessica shares her trauma story and how she was impacted by the discovery of her husband's sexual addiction.[2]

In my mind, I am sitting in that field of grass. Jesus, I know You are near.
You have opened my eyes, removed my mask, and revealed to me the pain I endured.
I see my wounds, I'm aware of my scars; I do not need to hide what You can see.
I cared for myself less than You care for me.
I grieve what was lost, say goodbye to the past.
I accept what You have for me, a new life without a mask.
Now, I walk forward, with You by my side.
I no longer have anything to hide.

Jessica's poem and the picture Jesus gave her was a prophetic promise to seal the healing He had worked in her life.

---

[2] Rebecca Bradley and Diane Roberts, *Behind the Mask* (Gresham: Pure Desire Ministries International, 2012), 171.

✚ How does this poem speak to you ?

_____

_____

_____

_____

_____

_____

_____

_____

_____

_____

Jessica realized that deep healing took place as she meditated on the prophetic promises God gave her. This will be true for you as you end this journey with your Betrayal & Beyond group and continue to meditate on God's personal promises to you.

Remember, this is the beginning of a new adventure, one you yourself can orchestrate for continued healing and growth. In these last two lessons, there are two more steps that will help in preparation for your new life and your next adventure.

Step One
CREATE A GOAL FOR A HEALTHY LIVING – A NEW NORMAL

In creating a goal for healthy living, think through all the things you have accomplished and changes you have made to reinforce your healing from betrayal. Choosing a life of health can be challenging. In many ways, as challenging as it was for us to choose Christ and a Christlike way of living:

Jesus helps us understand how difficult this choice can be:

> _Then Jesus said to his disciples, "If any of you wants to be my follower, you must give up your own way, take up your cross, and follow me. If you try to hang on to your life, you will lose it. But if you give up your life for my sake, you will save it."_
>
> MATTHEW 16:24-25 (NLT)

✛ **When it comes to healing from betrayal, what one area are you trying to hang on to or are reluctant to give up?**

In Matthew 16, Jesus doesn't say, "...take up my cross," but rather, "...take up your cross..." His cross was to die for the sins of the world; this is obviously not your cross. When Jesus faced the cross it meant death; when we face our cross, it means life and abundance. The cross you are to take up is often found where you're trying to hang on to things in your life that interfere with God's plan for your life. Jesus is saying to you, "The part of your life that is not working, the part of your life that causes you pain, if you will surrender this part of your life to Me, I have a gift for you. I can reach into this point of pain and trauma and heal you."

You will be able to hear these words clearly when you understand that every interaction with God is encased in grace. This is why the Holy Spirit gets so excited about what God wants to give you; He is excited because the gift God gives you is victory over the enemy and healing for your heart, mind, and soul.

Remember, because you are a follower of Christ, the enemy has nothing but contempt for you. Look at what he said about Job and all of mankind in the Old Testament.

> *Satan answered, "A human would do anything to save his life. But what do you think would happen if you reached down and took away his health? He'd curse you to your face, that's what."*
>
> JOB 2:4-5 (MSG)

✚ Draw a picture showing how the enemy's schemes have tried to destroy your relationship through betrayal. Show what he has used as weapons against you.

Satan is totally convinced that, when push comes to shove, self-preservation will always rule in the hearts of men and women. He sees us as creatures completely dominated by fear, solely directed by our desire to survive. The enemy has no way to predict what you will do if you aren't being compelled by your pain and trauma. Satan is helpless against a woman who has found healing from betrayal and is an empowering testament to others.

As you think about how you have prevailed in your healing, what weapons have you developed to use against the enemy?

- Trusting God's plan and purpose for your life, even if you can't see it now.
- Allow God's Word to reign in your life as a source of truth, hope, and healing.
- Obeying God, despite the difficulties you are going through.
- Doing what is right and pleasing to the Lord, despite the consequences.
- Choosing not to be controlled by pain and trauma, but instead accepting God's grace in your healing.

✚ **Which of the above statements have been most helpful and healing throughout this process? Explain.**

_____

_____

_____

_____

_____

_____

_____

_____

_____

_____

_____

God has given us promises about being overcomers, which are accessed when we are obedient to the Cross. Part of creating a goal for healthy living requires us to identify the fiery darts the enemy has been using against us in the form of thoughts, feelings, and relationship difficulties.

> _...above all, taking the shield of faith with which you will be able to quench all the fiery darts of the wicked one._
>
> EPHESIANS 6:16 (NKJV)

Allow the Holy Spirit to guide you with His wisdom and direct you in how to move in faith. Remember, choosing to walk in obedience to the Cross disarms the enemy.

✚ In the following table, identify the fiery darts the enemy has been using against you and the healthy strategies you can use as a shield of protection: as your obedience to the Cross.

DEFEATING THE ASSAULTS OF THE ENEMY

The Enemy's Fiery Darts	Your Obedience to the Cross
You will never be able to fully trust your husband; you can never let him out of your sight.	*I have a Safety Action Plan I will follow and women who will continue to support me through this process*
You're disqualified from ministry because your own family fell apart.	*God will equip me to offer comfort and hope to women who have experienced betrayal; the same comfort and hope God gave me.*

_____

_____

_____

_____

_____

_____

_____

_____

Having a clear goal in life is crucial to our lifelong healing from betrayal. Setting healthy boundaries and having a good sense of self-assertiveness allows women to make healthy choices as they continue on their healing journey. Self-assertiveness is a characteristic that shows you respect yourself by the way you stand up for your own interests, express your thoughts and feelings in a healthy way, and value yourself enough to invest in your holistic health. How do we develop a healthy sense of self-assertiveness? Long term self-care is key.

LONG TERM SELF-CARE

Developing a long term self-care plan may be challenging. Many women realize they have been neglecting themselves for decades, so changing the focus on personal care seems strange and almost selfish. However, there is only one you and only you can keep yourself healthy and growing. Throughout this journey, we hope you have become more in touch with your needs, wants, hopes, and dreams. We trust it will be the foundational work of your new life, one in which you utilize helpful tools, new knowledge, and hard-won ground in your transformation.

As you work on developing a long term care plan, consider the following ideas.[3] Hopefully, many will become part of your daily routines. Take some time and decide what you need to be doing for yourself.

- Deep breathing and meditation/worship to increase oxygen levels in the brain and become better in tune with yourself and centered on Christ.

_____

[3] Jane Carter, one of my original leaders for Betrayal & Beyond, put together this self-care information.

- Surround yourself with hope-filled messages through the books you read, music you hear, media you enjoy, and friends and groups with which you interact.
- Regular exercise to increase blood flow and body strength, as well as to release muscle tension.
- Regular interaction with healthy friends for problem solving, validation, encouragement, and prayer.
- Create new, healthy behaviors to nurture yourself; on your own or with family and friends.
- Incorporate more creative/right-brained activities into your daily life for greater joy and health (e.g. singing, fine arts, dance, crafts, music, writing).
- Journal regularly to increase your connection with God and yourself.
- Use the Double Bind exercise when faced with a difficult decision: to look at options, solve issues, and keep moving toward health.
- Get good sleep to rejuvenate and heal the body and brain.
- Avoid toxic substances (e.g., drugs, cigarettes, excessive alcohol, caffeine, fast food, refined sugars and flours) and toxic attitudes (e.g., bitterness, rage, unforgiveness, pride, hopelessness, helplessness).
- Obtain counseling to work through trauma issues.
- Ask your doctor about the potential need for taking specific medications to help you get balanced and improve daily functioning.
- After completing this group, consider co-leading the next group.
- Take other classes to work on specific areas that need healing.
- _____
- _____
- _____

✛ **Which of the above self-care suggestions would you like to implement into your goal for healthy living?**

_____

_____

_____

_____

_____

_____

Seeing God's Redemption Through the Pain

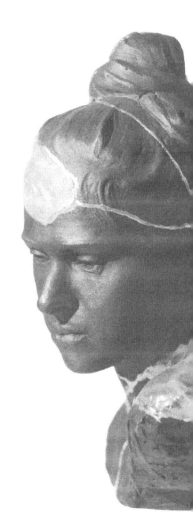

There is an aspect to this process that shows up at some point in a partner's healing journey: purpose. When we begin to see that although this has been a painful journey, even excruciating at times, God has had purpose in all of this: to bring about His will and His glory in our lives.

> *He has saved us and called us to a holy life—not because of anything we have done but because of his own purpose and grace.*
>
> 2 TIMOTHY 1:9 (NIV)

What does it mean to have purpose? We often think of purpose as the reason something exists or the intended result or outcome of something. And it is our perceived purpose that gives meaning and direction to various areas of our life. In many ways, purpose becomes our guide; helping us stay focused on what we want to achieve and driving us toward our goals.

For many partners, when discovery or disclosure happens, they lose their sense of purpose. It's as though betrayal sucked all the wind from their sails, and they are left stranded and motionless in the ocean. But after they have worked on healing from the effects of betrayal, they find new meaning and purpose. This newfound purpose is life-giving and empowers a stronger wind in their sails, because it comes from God's grace and healing in their lives. They are fearless as they set sail toward their new life and next adventure.

✚ When did you begin to see God's purpose in your healing from betrayal?

_____

_____

_____

_____

✚ What parts of your healing experience have strengthened and empowered you to keep moving toward health?

_____

_____

_____

_____

In the last lesson, we talked about the final two steps that will help in preparation for your new life and next adventure. Step one was: Create a Goal for a Healthy Living—a New Normal.

Step Two
DISCOVER YOUR DREAMS

In this new season of being a grandparent, our family is often treated to some kind of performance by one or more of our four grandchildren. It is amazing how young children can create entertainment for us that includes song, dance, and even taekwondo all in one performance. Recently, one of our granddaughters was dancing around the family room and Ted asked, "Are you my little ballerina?" She turned and looked at grandpa as if he was clueless and emphatically stated, "I'm a prima ballerina!" At age seven she was dreaming of herself as the main star of a ballet company.

✝ **Share some of the dreams you had as a child.**

_____

_____

_____

_____

Children have the capacity to see the possibilities and dream without limits. God placed this in all of us. Sometimes our dreams and desires give way to conformity and we put on masks, adapting ourselves to the expectations of others, real or imagined. Or we allow life's pain and trauma to chase away our dreams.

Maybe you stopped dreaming even before you discovered the betrayal. Or maybe you have experienced such devastating consequences from your husband's betrayal, you have given up on your dreams.

Let's look at God's Word in Jeremiah 29:11, cited here in two translations:

> _For I know the thoughts that I think toward you, says the LORD, thoughts of peace and not of evil, to give you a future and a hope. (NKJV)_
>
> _I'll show up and take care of you as I promised and bring you back home. I know what I'm doing. I have it all planned out—plans to take care of you, not abandon you, plans to give you the future you hope for. (MSG)_

Jeremiah is writing to a people who are in exile and whose nation would be ravaged and destroyed. Yet he declares this stunning promise in the midst of their captivity. He tells them (in verses 4-7) that even though they were carried away and this was not of their own doing, they should go on living, build houses and plant gardens and eat of their fruit. He even challenges them to pray for their captors.

✝ **In what way(s) are you encouraged by Jeremiah 29:11? How does it give you hope for your future?**

_____

_____

_____

_____

You are at a crossroads in your life. You have gone through the *Betrayal & Beyond Workbook* and Journal, and have processed some of your pain and trauma created by betrayal. You have received the support of others who are on a similar journey. And now you have to decide to move forward, regardless of where your marriage is today.

In earlier lessons, we shared how God takes all that the enemy has used to discourage and destroy us and He uses it for His glory. He makes beauty out of ashes. We know this is true because we see it in Scripture.

Sometimes it is hard to see because God is good at hiding treasures in unusual places:

- He hid a warrior inside a shepherd boy named David; even Goliath was surprised.
- He hid a deliverer of His people inside a fugitive murderer named Moses.
- He hid a queen who delivered His people inside an orphaned Jewish girl named Esther.
- He hid a King and Savior inside a boy of humble birth.

✚ **What has God hidden inside you ?**

_____

_____

_____

_____

_____

> *But we have this treasure in earthen vessels, that the excellence of the power may be of God and not of us.*
>
> 2 CORINTHIANS 4:7 (NKJV)

What a paradox of how God can take weak human beings and use them for instruments of power in this world! God has created in each of us talents, treasures, and divine dreams that can be a legacy for others.

God has given you gifts in the past and present.

To understand God's future plans for you, it's important to take an inventory of your victories, talents, and gifts, both past and present.

The following exercise will help you think through what God might be saying to you about your accomplishments, your dreams, and your purpose. The chart will help you identify the victories and events that were impactful, how you were able to use your talents and gifts, and relationships that have been significant to you.

✚ Write the answers from your life in the following chart.

THE GIFTS GOD HAS GIVEN ME FROM MY PAST AND PRESENT

Past and Present Victories and Events	Use of Talents and Gifts	Relationships built from these experiences
Auditioned for drama and got a part in a play.	I used my drama skills in putting on productions in our church.	I met some lifelong friends by being a part of the various drama teams.
Joined and excelled on the school debate team.	Developed my skills of speaking to an audience.	Debate team coach believed in me and encouraged my speaking gifts.
This is my second time through Betrayal & Beyond.	I was a co-leader and want to lead my own group now.	I have maintained close ties to my original leader and the women in that group.

✚ **What patterns do you notice about your gifts, talents, experiences, or relationships? What traits, talents, or unique gifts might be present in you for His glory?**

Example: *Public speaking and leading others is one of my passions.*

Example: *I have worked through my own healing from betrayal and want to help other women find healing.*

_____

_____

_____

_____

_____

_____

_____

_____

_____

_____

_____

YOUR LEGACY: GIFTS FOR OTHERS

As you begin to think about your legacy to your children, grandchildren, and others whose lives you have and will touch, consider this poem entitled, "The Dash" by Linda Ellis.[4] It poses the question: How will you live your dash? It asks you to imagine your tombstone with your birth date—(dash)—and then the date of your death. Only those who knew and loved you "know what that little line is worth." What will be remembered is not how many material things you have or your social status, but rather "how you lived and loved and how you spent your dash."

How will you finish what is left of your "dash?"

In light of the treasures God has created in you, what is the legacy He wants you to give others? Ask Him what He has in mind for the remaining years you have on this earth.

---

[4] Linda Ellis, *The Dash*, 1996. To see the complete text of the poem or for more information about the author, see www.lindaslyrics.com.

✝ Draw a picture of what gifts God might have you leave for others. Use words, pictures, symbols, or whatever comes to mind as you listen to what God is speaking to you through His Holy Spirit.

✚ Write a brief description of what you have drawn.

_____

_____

_____

_____

_____

_____

✚ Personalize a prayer in light of the talents and gifts God has given you.
(You can use this prayer as a template to write your own prayer.)

Lord,

*Thank you for the talents, treasures, and dreams You have created in me. You know how I began and when my life will end; my time is in Your hands. I want to make the most of the rest of my "**dash**" and with Your help, I want to leave a legacy that glorifies You. Open my heart for all You have for me that I might experience the abundant life You have promised. May my life of love for You and surrender to Your purpose be a source of blessing and a rich legacy for my family, my friends, and my descendants.*

_____

_____

_____

_____

_____

_____

Note: If you are feeling triggered by any of the lesson content or this healing process, and want to pursue professional help, please contact Pure Desire at 503-489-0230 or visit **puredesire.org/counseling**; or contact APSATS (The Association of Partners of Sex Addicts Trauma Specialists) at 513-874-2342 or email **info@apsats.org**.

Congratulations!

Although you have just finished walking through probably one of the most difficult journeys in your life, we at Pure Desire know that God will bless your efforts. Women who have traveled before you have said that while it was the most painful season of their life, it was also the most rewarding season. We pray you will see much fruit and continued healing from your investment in walking through this *Workbook*. We also pray you will see yourself in light of who God says you are and what you have accomplished so far. Be assured, this is just the beginning of what God wants to do in you and through you as you complete the rest of your "dash."

Next Steps

Over the past several months, you have transformed and developed a new way of doing life. You have become more emotionally aware. You have implemented strategies that have empowered you to keep moving forward in your healing. And, as you have walked this journey together, you have created relationships with the women in your group. These relationships don't have to end here.

Although your group has ended, we encourage you to get together four weeks after your last group meeting and check in. See where everyone is at and if anyone needs support in taking their next step.

The work you have done throughout this journey is only the beginning. It is the foundation on which your next steps are built:

- Go through *Betrayal & Beyond* again, if your healing still feels "in process."
- Consider leading or co-leading a Betrayal & Beyond group, either in your church or online.
  - ▷ For training to become a group leader, visit **puredesire.org/glt**.
  - ▷ For info on bringing PD to your church, visit **puredesire.org/group-pathway**
- If you struggle with unprocessed love, sex, and relationship issues, consider joining an Unraveled group.

Also, if God has used this ministry and *Betrayal & Beyond* to change your life, would you consider helping others find hope, healing, and freedom by joining Team 58? This is a group of men and women dedicated to supporting the work of Pure Desire through recurring monthly donations. To learn more about Team 58, visit **puredesire.org/give**.

Whatever you decide to do, keep moving forward. It is through this forward motion that we continue to learn and change and grow.

This is how we step into the life God created us for.

> **This is how we become the woman God created us to be.**

Appendix

Primary, Secondary, and Tertiary Emotions

This chart can help us understand how many of our initial emotions have deeper, underlying feelings. These secondary and tertiary emotions may be the true root feeling and yet masked by the primary emotion for various reasons. This is not an all-inclusive list, but may help you better identify your own depth of emotions.

Primary	Secondary	Tertiary
Love	Affection	Adoration, affection, love, fondness, liking, attraction, caring, tenderness, compassion, sentimentality
	Lust	Arousal, desire, lust, passion, infatuation
	Longing	Longing
Joy	Cheerfulness	Amusement, bliss, cheerfulness, gaiety, glee, jolliness, joviality, joy, delight, enjoyment, gladness, happiness, jubilation, elation, satisfaction, euphoria
	Zest	Enthusiasm, zeal, zest, excitement, thrill, exhilaration
	Contentment	Contentment, pleasure
	Pride	Pride, triumph
	Optimism	Eagerness, hope, optimism
	Enthrallment	Enthrallment, rapture
	Relief	Relief

Surprise	Surprise	Amazement, surprise, astonishment
Anger	Irritation	Aggravation, irritation, agitation, annoyance, grouchiness, grumpiness
	Exasperation	Exasperation, frustration
	Rage	Anger, rage, outrage, fury, wrath, hostility, ferocity, bitterness, hate, scorn, spite, vengefulness, dislike, resentment
	Disgust	Disgust, revulsion, contempt, loathing
	Envy	Envy, jealousy
	Torment	Torment
Sadness	Suffering	Agony, suffering, hurt, anguish
	Sadness	Depression, despair, hopelessness, gloom, glumness, sadness, unhappiness, grief, sorrow, woe, misery, melancholy
	Disappointment	Dismay, disappointment, displeasure
	Shame	Guild, shame, regret, remorse
	Neglect	Alienation, isolation, neglect, loneliness, rejection, homesickness, defeat, dejection, insecurity, embarrassment, humiliation, insult
	Sympathy	Pity, sympathy
Fear	Horror	Alarm, shock, fear, fright, horror, terror, panic, hysteria, mortification
	Nervousness	Anxiety, nervousness, tenseness, uneasiness, apprehension, worry, distress, dread

The Feeling Wheel⁵

Exploring our feelings during a healing process is often difficult, especially if we have been raised, taught, or encouraged to ignore our feelings. Many times, we recognize we are sad, mad, or scared. Additionally, this chart helps uncover our feelings beyond the surface of sad, mad, or scared, and acknowledge the underlying and opposing emotion. For example, the color opposite sad (negative) is joy (positive). God's heart for us is that we would begin to understand and process all our feelings, clearing a path to begin experiencing not only the richness of our feelings, but expanding our awareness of our feelings.

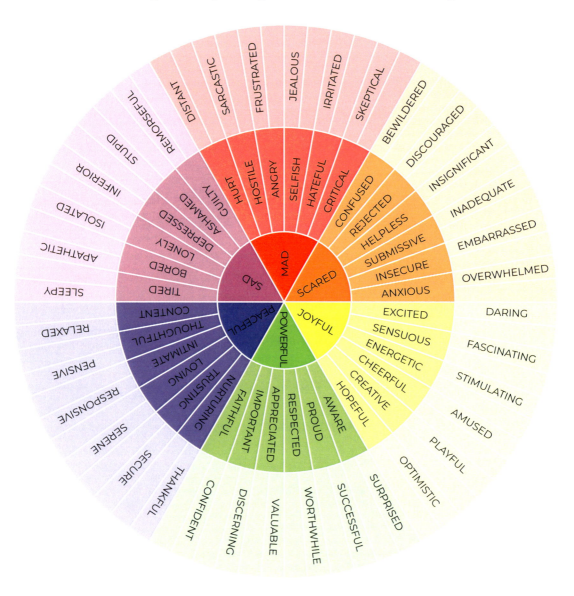

---

⁵ Willcox, G. (1982). The Feeling Wheel: A Tool for Expanding Awareness of Emotions and Increasing Spontaneity and Intimacy. *Transactional Analysis Journal, 12*(4), 274–276.

Alphabetized Emotions

Abandoned
Adequate
Adamant
Affectionate
Agitated
Agony
Almighty
Ambivalent
Angry
Annoyed
Anxious
Apathetic
Astounded
Awed
Awkward
Bad
Beautiful
Betrayed
Bitter
Blissful
Bold
Bored
Bothered
Burdened
Calm
Capable
Captivated
Challenged
Charmed
Cheated
Cheerful
Cherished
Childish
Childlike
Clever
Combative
Competent
Competitive
Compulsive
Condemned
Confused
Conspicuous
Contented
Contrite
Crazy
Cruel
Crushed
Culpable

Deceitful
Defeated
Delighted
Depleted
Desirous
Despair
Destructive
Determined
Different
Diffident
Diminished
Discontented
Disgusted
Distracted
Distraught
Disturbed
Divided
Dominated
Dubious
Eager
Ecstatic
Electrified
Empty
Enchanted
Energetic
Enjoyment
Enraptured
Envious
Evil
Exasperated
Excited
Exhausted
Fascinated
Fawning
Fearful
Flustered
Foolish
Frantic
Free
Frenzied
Frightened
Frustrated
Full
Furious
Generous
Glad
Good
Grateful

Gratified
Greedy
Grief
Guilty
Gullible
Happy
Harassed
Hate
Heavenly
Helpful
Helpless
High
Homesick
Honored
Hopeful
Horrible
Hurt
Hysterical
Ignorant
Ignored
Immoral
Imposed upon
Impressed
Infatuated
Infuriated
Inspired
Intimidated
Isolated
Jealous
Joyous
Judgmental
Jumpy
Kind
Laconic
Lazy
Lecherous
Left out
Liberated
Lonely
Longing
Lost
Lovely
Loving
Low
Lustful
Mad
Mean
Melancholy

Miserable
Naive
Naughty
Neglected
Nervous
Nice
Nutty
Obnoxious
Obsessed
Odd
Opposed
Outraged
Overwhelmed
Pain
Panicked
Parsimonious
Peaceful
Persecuted
Petrified
Pity
Pleasant
Pleased
Precarious
Pressured
Pretty
Prim
Prissy
Proud
Quarrelsome
Rage
Refreshed
Rejected
Relaxed
Relieved
Remorse
Restless
Reverent
Rewarded
Righteous
Sad
Satisfied
Scared
Screwed up
Self-righteous
Servile
Settled
Sexy
Shocked

Silly
Skeptical
Small
Sneaky
Soft
Solemn
Sorrowful
Spiteful
Startled
Stingy
Stuffed
Stunned
Stupefied
Suffering
Sure
Sympathetic
Talkative
Teary
Tempted
Tenacious
Tense
Tentative
Tenuous
Terrible
Terrified
Threatened
Thwarted
Tired
Trapped
Troubled
Trusting
Ugly
Uneasy
Unimportant
Unsettled
Vehement
Violent
Vital
Vivacious
Vulnerable
Weary
Weepy
Wholesome
Wicked
Wonderful
Worried
Zany
Zestful

What a Polygraph Can and Cannot Do

The polygraph test is a tool that can be used to begin to restore trust in a relationship. It can be given within 30 days of disclosure or discovery and can be followed up every 90 days with another polygraph test to ensure greater accountability. If trust begins to grow, you may want to repeat the test every six months, and then one every year, depending upon the type of addiction.

Most sex addicts don't like the idea of a polygraph test because they've never had their behavior measured objectively. But over time, we have found that individuals who are serious about recovery actually see this as a helpful measure of how they are moving toward health. Also, when they know there will be a follow-up test, it encourages them to think twice about returning to old patterns.

A polygraph test cannot guarantee that he will not lie again or that he will stop his addictive behavior, but it can promote safety and trust. Although this tool can help to reestablish trust, the goal is to eventually leave the tool behind and begin to trust based on a growing intimacy in the relationship.

CAUTION!

There are a few cautions we give to partners who have requested this test:

- Be careful that the polygraph is not used to feed your need for validation, vindication, or to be a detective.

- If your husband passes, don't challenge the test. If you have concerns, wait until the next polygraph test. If there are inconsistencies in his behavior, expect them to be revealed in the next polygraph test.

FULL DISCLOSURE POLYGRAPH TESTS

The most effective polygraph tests are "full disclosure polygraphs" which take between two and three hours initially. We recommend you use a CSAT (Certified Sex Addition Therapist) during this process (visit puredesire.org/program-overview/ for information regarding Full Disclosure Counseling). Many of the Pure Desire counselors can help you through this process via secure video conferencing. The addict will need to submit a detailed sexual history of his sexual behaviors as far back as he can remember up to present day. It will include all sexual behavior outside the marriage. The counselor will look it over to make sure nothing is left out. The addict takes his full sexual history and 3-5 questions from his wife to the polygraph examiner, who will ask him questions in light of those two documents.

You can find a "polygraph examiner," through an online search or check with local attorneys who can put you in contact with someone who can give a "full disclosure polygraph." Our Pure Desire office also has polygraphers we can recommend and a written statement to the polygrapher that explains the purpose of the polygraph.

WHAT DO I DO WITH THE RESULTS?

It is best to have the results sent to a counselor who can debrief you as a couple.

QUESTIONS FOR THE POLYGRAPH TEST

The polygraph examiner will need 3-5 "yes or no" questions submitted by the wife in a sealed envelope. This allows the wife to get answers to specific questions she might have.

The following suggestions will help you write out your own personal questions that can be included in the polygraph. Because many partners have no idea what to ask, we have provided some examples. The comments in parenthesis give you options with specific time frames: since we have been married, since we started counseling, since you joined a Pure Desire group.

Note: If you are asking questions about sex with minors, find out ahead of time if the examiner is a mandatory reporter. If they learn that children are at risk, by law, and in most cases, they must report these findings, which can lead to criminal charges.

01. Have you had sexual contact with another woman during the course of our marriage? If so, have you had more than one? If so, do I know her? If so, do you still have contact with this person through a social or work environment or social media?

02. Have you gone looking or cruising where prostitutes hang out during the course of our marriage? Have you had sexual contact with a prostitute? Have you visited topless bars or strip clubs?

03. Have you paid for and received sexual favors from anyone, male or female, during the course of our marriage?

04. Have you ever had a physical or sexual relationship with another man? Have you ever had physical or sexual contact with a man more than once?

05. In the course of our marriage (or since we started Pure Desire groups/counseling) have you used the Internet with the intent to act out sexually? Have you used the TV to act out sexually? Have you used movies to act out sexually? Have you used the cell phone to act out sexually?

06. Have you used masturbation to meet your sexual needs during our marriage (or since we started counseling, or since you joined a Pure Desire group)? Have you used masturbation more than once a week to meet your sexual needs during the course of our marriage?

07. Have you been totally honest about all these issues with your wife? Have you been totally honest with your men's group that you are accountable to and/or your counselor?

08. As an adult, have you had sexual contact with children? (Caution! The answers to this question could lead to criminal charges.)

Recommended Reading

PURE DESIRE BOOKS:

Peace Beyond the Tears, by Tina Harris

Connected: Building a Bridge to Intimacy, by Tyler Chinchen, Harry Flanagan, Diane Roberts, and Ted Roberts

OTHER BOOKS:

Boundaries in Marriage, by Henry Cloud and John Townsend

From Betrayal Trauma to Healing & Joy, by Marsha Means

Help Her Heal: An Empathy Workbook for Sex Addicts to Help their Partners Heal, by Carol Juergensen Sheets and Allan J. Katz

Intimate Deception, by Sheri Keffer

Mending a Shattered Heart, by Stefanie Carnes

Partner Betrayal Trauma, by Douglas Weiss

The Body Keeps the Score, by Bessel van der Kolk

The Gift of Sex, by Clifford Penner and Joyce Penner

The Great Sex Rescue, by Sheila Wray Gregoire

Treating Trauma from Sexual Betrayal, by Kevin Skinner

Worthy of Her Trust, by Stephen Arterburn and Jason Martinkus

Your Sexually Addicted Spouse, by Barbara Steffens and Marsha Means

Sexual Integrity 101

When it comes to understanding the impact of sexual brokenness and betrayal trauma, *Sexual Integrity 101* can help! This 8-week video course provides an expansive view of the factors that contribute to unwanted sexual behaviors and how the recovery journey leads to hope, healing, and freedom. Loaded with foundational teaching, interviews with experts in the field of sexual health, and testimonies from those transformed through a safe, grace-filled process, it will give you practical tools and strategies that lead to lasting health. This video training is for men, women, students, pastors, lay leaders, parents, and more. It's for anyone who wants to find freedom from the effects of unwanted sexual behaviors and betrayal trauma.

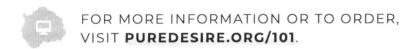

FOR MORE INFORMATION OR TO ORDER,
VISIT **PUREDESIRE.ORG/101**.

Group Leader Training

If you have a heart for helping others find healing, the *Group Leader Training* course was designed to equip men and women to lead an effective, life-changing group. This course reflects a combined knowledge of over 30 years of leading Pure Desire groups. It takes the best practices, tips, and tools Pure Desire offers and packages it ALL in one place. It covers topics like Pure Desire's approach to running groups, how to promote groups, the disclosure process, handling challenging group members and problem situations, facing legal issues, and more!

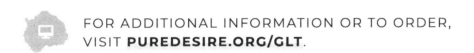

FOR ADDITIONAL INFORMATION OR TO ORDER,
VISIT **PUREDESIRE.ORG/GLT**.